Top 100 Baby Purees

Also by Annabel Karmel

The Fussy Eaters' Recipe Book

Lunch Boxes and Snacks

Complete Party Planner

SuperFoods

Favorite Family Meals

The Healthy Baby Meal Planner

Annabel Karmel
Top 100 Baby Purees

100 quick and easy meals for a healthy and happy baby

ATRIA BOOKS

New York   London   Toronto   Sydney

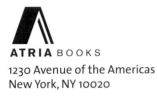

ATRIA BOOKS

1230 Avenue of the Americas
New York, NY 10020

Library of Congress Cataloging-in-Publication Data
Karmel, Annabel.
    Top 100 baby purees : 100 quick and easy meals for a healthy and happy baby / Annabel Karmel.
        p.   cm.
    Includes index.
    1. Cookery (Baby foods).   2. Infants—Nutrition.   I. Title.
TX740.K293   2006
641.5'6222—dc22   2005059103

ISBN-13: 978-0-7432-8957-3
ISBN-10:   0-7432-8957-9

First Atria Books hardcover edition March 2006

20

ATRIA BOOKS is a trademark of Simon & Schuster, Inc.

Manufactured in China

For information about special discounts for bulk purchases,
please contact Simon & Schuster Special Sales:
1-800-456-6798 or business@simonandschuster.com.

Contents

PREFACE by Michel Cohen, M.D. 6

INTRODUCTION
Starting solids 7
Food allergies 12
Weaning preterm babies 18

FIRST-STAGE WEANING: 6 MONTHS 21

AFTER FIRST TASTES: 6 TO 7 MONTHS 33

SECOND-STAGE WEANING: 7 TO 9 MONTHS 63

GROWING INDEPENDENCE: 9 TO 12 MONTHS 97

BASICS 124

INDEX 127

ACKNOWLEDGMENTS 128

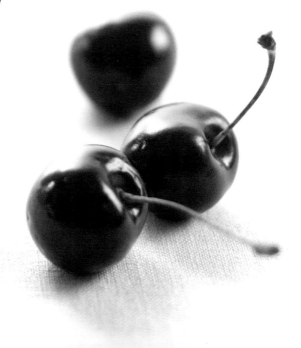

Preface

Why bother with making baby food? What's wrong with baby food from a jar, anyway? Take one of those jars and look carefully at the expiration date. The substance inside has been designed to last for two years past the date of purchase. That's not exactly the fresh food that you intended to feed your baby. But that's not the worst of it. At their best, commercial baby foods are bland and tasteless. In most cases, they're simply unappealing. How can children develop any sense of taste if they start out with foods that don't have any?

I have seen countless parents of ten-month-old babies who complain about their child's lack of interest in new foods, when in fact what they're really witnessing is their baby's determination to avoid eating any of these unctuous, flavorless purees. The second six months of life is the only window of opportunity you have to develop your baby's taste buds. If you miss this precious time, your child may join the ranks of picky eaters simply because of a lack of exposure to interesting, delicious food.

There is nothing wrong with giving babies prepared foods for the sake of convenience, but don't believe these preparations are a healthier option. The healthiest baby foods are the ones you make yourself. The result will certainly be fresher and far tastier than anything manufactured by a giant baby-food corporation.

To help you in this, *Top 100 Baby Purees* offers a wealth of resources for you to start making food for your baby. In an enjoyable way, you will learn how to introduce a variety of nutritious foods and seasonings that you never thought your baby would like. I guarantee you will get applause and big smiles. Most of all, you will put your baby and your family on the road to good health by offering balanced nutrition and creating healthy eating habits.

Michel Cohen, M.D., author of *The New Basics: A–to–Z Baby & Child Care for the Modern Parent*

Introduction

Starting solids

Babies grow more rapidly in their first year than at any other time in their life, so how you feed your newborn will be one of the most important decisions you make for your new baby.

Don't be in a hurry to wean your baby onto solids. For the first six months or so, breast milk or formula provides all the nutrients your baby needs, and should remain the main source of nourishment. Breast-feeding exclusively is recommended for this period.

At around six months, however, your baby will reach a stage where she needs solid foods as well as milk in her diet. For example, the store of iron that she will have been born with will have been used up, so it will be important to include iron-rich foods in her diet (see page 8).

There is no "right" age at which to introduce solids, though, as every baby is different. However, solids should not be introduced before seventeen weeks after your child is born. A young baby's digestive system is not sufficiently developed before this time and there is a greater risk of allergy developing. If you feel that your baby needs solids earlier than at six months, speak to your pediatrician or GP.

Signs that your baby is ready:
• still hungry after a full milk feeding
• demands feedings more frequently
• wakes at night for a feeding previously slept through

Your baby's nutritional needs

The nutritional needs of babies and toddlers are different from those of adults—a low-fat, high-fiber diet is good for a full-grown person but not appropriate for babies or young children, as they need more fat and concentrated sources of calories and nutrients to fuel their rapid growth. With this in mind, it is best not to give low-fat dairy products, such as milk and yogurt, to young children, but choose instead the full-fat variety.

Neither should they be given too much fiber, as it tends to be bulky and can fill them up before they take in all the nutrients they need for proper growth and development. In addition, excess fiber can flush out valuable minerals and cause other problems such as diarrhea. Consequently, fibrous foods like dried fruits, beans, and peas should be given in moderation, as should whole-wheat bread and whole-grain cereals like shredded wheat. Likewise, fruit purees, such as apple, pear, and plum, shouldn't be given too frequently.

Babies should eat a wide variety of fruit and vegetables, however, to ensure they have plenty of vitamins and minerals in their diet. After the first few weeks of weaning, make sure that, as well as fruit and vegetable purees, you give foods that are relatively high in calories, such as mashed avocado, fruit mixed with yogurt, or Vegetables with Cheese Sauce (see pages 30, 55, and 71).

Iron is very important for your baby's mental and physical development. A baby is born with a store of iron that lasts for about six months. After that, it is important that your baby gets the iron she needs from her diet. Iron in foods of animal origin, like red meat or poultry, is much better absorbed than iron in foods of plant origin, like green vegetables or cereal. Vitamin C helps boost iron absorption, so give your baby vitamin C–rich fruits like berry or citrus fruits (but not before six months—see page 9), or vegetables like broccoli or sweet pepper.

Vitamin supplements

For most babies vitamin supplements are probably unnecessary, so long as they are eating fresh food in sufficient quantity and drinking formula milk until the age of one. However, government health agencies have recommended that if your baby is being breast-fed (breast milk doesn't contain enough vitamin D) or is drinking less than 18 ounces of infant formula a day, you should give your baby vitamin supplements from six months to two years of age. Ask your pediatrician for advice.

The benefits of homemade baby food

The ingredients of most commercial baby foods have been heated to a very high temperature and then cooled, in order to sterilize them. This gives them a very long shelf life (usually two years) but destroys a lot of the flavor and some of the nutrients in the process. There is nothing better for your baby than making your own fresh baby food, and it is cheaper than buying the commercial variety. You will know exactly what the ingredients are, you can introduce a wide range of foods, and your baby will get used to eating like the rest of the family so the transition to family meals will be easier. Preparing larger quantities than you need and freezing small portions in ice-cube trays or small containers can save you time and effort.

The importance of milk in a baby's diet

As stated above, breast or formula milk should provide all the nutrients your baby needs in the first six months. Ideally, you should try to breast-feed your baby until he is at least six months (twenty-six weeks) old. Indeed, it's best not to give your baby anything except breast milk during that period. Even after your baby starts eating other foods, it is still really important to make sure he gets enough milk. Between six months and one year, babies should still be receiving a minimum of 18 ounces of breast or formula milk a day.

Breast milk is always preferable to formula because, in addition to meeting all of your baby's nutritional requirements, it contains antibodies that will help your baby fight illness and infection. Breast-feeding for six months has also been shown to delay the onset and reduce the severity of allergies in children from families with a history of asthma, hay fever, eczema, and food allergy.

You should continue to give breast or formula milk to your baby as his main drink for the entire first year, as cow's milk does not contain enough iron or other nutrients for proper growth. However, from six months full-fat cow's milk can be used in cooking—for example, when making a cheese sauce for your baby—and can also be given with his breakfast cereal.

The best first foods for your baby

Very first foods should be easy to digest and unlikely to provoke an allergic reaction. I find that root vegetables like CARROT, SWEET POTATO, PARSNIP, and RUTABAGA tend to go down best with very young babies due to these vegetables' naturally sweet flavor and smooth texture once pureed. APPLE and PEAR make good first fruit purees. BANANA and PAPAYA do not require cooking, provided they are ripe, and can be pureed or mashed on their own, or together, with a little breast or formula milk. It's important that you choose fruits that are ripe and have a good flavor, so it's best to taste them yourself first before giving them to your baby.

Another good first food is BABY RICE CEREAL. Mixed with water or breast or formula milk, it's easily digested, and its milky taste makes for an easy transition to solids. Choose one that is sugar free and enriched with vitamins and iron. Baby rice also combines well with both fruit and vegetable purees.

Foods to avoid

BERRY and CITRUS FRUITS, including fruit juice like orange and lemon juice, can trigger a reaction but rarely cause a true allergy. They can be given from six months.

FISH and SHELLFISH should not be given before six months due to the risk of food poisoning and potential allergy.

HONEY should not be given before one year. Very occasionally honey can contain a type of bacteria that can result in a potentially serious illness known as infant botulism. After a baby is a year old, the intestine matures and the bacteria can't grow, so giving honey at that stage is no problem.

NUTS and SEEDS, including peanuts, peanut butter, and other nut spreads, should be strictly avoided if there is any risk of allergic reaction, such as a family history. Peanut butter and nut spreads can be given from six months provided there is no history of allergy in the family. Whole nuts of any kind are not recommended before the age of five due to the risk of choking.

RAW or LIGHTLY COOKED EGGS should be strictly

avoided due to the risk of salmonella infection. Eggs should not be given before six months and should be cooked until the yolk and white are solid.

SALT: Babies under a year should not have any salt added to their food, as this can strain immature kidneys and cause dehydration. A preference for salt can become established at an early age, and eating too much salt may lead to high blood pressure later in life. Babies up to six months old should have less than 1g salt (less than ¼ teaspoon) a day, and from seven months old they should have a maximum of 1g salt a day. Avoid giving your baby processed foods that are not made specifically for babies, such as pasta sauces and most breakfast cereals, because these can be high in salt. Likewise, smoked foods should be avoided because of their high salt content.

SUGAR: Unless food is really tart, don't add sugar. Adding sugar is habit forming and increases the risk of tooth decay when your baby's first teeth start to come through.

UNPASTEURIZED CHEESES, such as Brie, Camembert, or Danish Blue, should not be given before twelve months due to the risk of listeria infection.

WHEAT-BASED FOODS and other foods that contain GLUTEN—such as wheat, barley, and rye—should not be introduced before six months. When buying baby cereals and zwiebacks before six months, make sure they are gluten free. Baby rice is the safest type of cereal to try at first.

Cooking baby foods

BAKING: If you are cooking something in the oven for the whole family, you could take the opportunity to bake a potato, sweet potato, or butternut squash for your baby. Wash, prick the chosen vegetable with a fork, and bake in an oven preheated to 375°F for about 1 hour or until tender. Cut in half, scoop out the flesh, and mash together with a little milk and a pat of butter.

BOILING: Use the minimum amount of water— just enough to cover whatever is in the pan— and be careful not to overcook the vegetables, or the nutrients they contain will be lost. Add enough of the cooking liquid to the vegetables to make a smooth puree.

MICROWAVING: Chop the vegetables or fruit and place in a suitable dish. Add a little water, cover, leaving an air vent, and cook on full power until tender. Puree to the desired consistency but take care to stir well and check that it is not too hot to serve to your baby.

STEAMING is the best way to preserve the fresh taste and vitamins in vegetables and fruits. Vitamins B and C are water soluble and can easily be destroyed by overcooking, especially when fruits and vegetables are boiled. Broccoli loses over 60 percent of its antioxidants when boiled, for instance, but less than 7 percent when steamed. It's worth buying a multilayered steamer, which enables you to cook three different vegetables at once. When pureeing vegetables, you can add a little of the boiled water from the bottom of the steamer if the puree is not smooth enough.

STEWING: Put chopped fruit, such as peeled apples or pears, into a heavy-bottomed saucepan and, if necessary, add a little water or fruit juice. Cover and cook over low heat until tender, then blend the fruit to a puree. Spoon a little into your baby's bowl and serve lukewarm.

Pureeing

During the first few weeks of weaning, it is important that the food you offer your baby is smooth, not too thick, and never lumpy.

FOOD PROCESSOR: This is good for pureeing larger quantities, such as when making batches of purees for freezing. Many food processors have mini bowl attachments that will serve the purpose better when pureeing smaller quantities. The downside is that they involve more cleanup than handheld electric blenders. Pureeing potato in a food processor tends to break down the starches and produce a sticky, glutinous pulp, so it is much better to puree it using a food mill.

HANDHELD ELECTRIC BLENDER: This is ideal for making baby purees, especially in very small quantities.

FOOD MILL: This is turned by hand, and it is ideal for pureeing vegetables like potato or sweet potato. A food mill is also good for pureeing foods that have a tough skin, like peas or dried apricots, as you can discard the harder bits.

Freezing food

• Flexible plastic ice-cube trays are ideal for freezing baby food, but make sure that you seal these in freezer bags. Once frozen, knock out and store the cubes in well-sealed freezer bags and label with the contents and expiration date (see below).

• If you freeze food in ice-cube trays, you can defrost two individual flavors and mix them together to make combinations like apple and pear or sweet potato and parsnip.

• Never refreeze meals that have already been frozen. The exception to this is that raw frozen food can be returned to the freezer once it is cooked. For example, cooked frozen peas can be refrozen.

• Frozen baby purees will keep for six weeks.

• When batch-cooking, cool food as quickly as possible and then freeze it. Don't leave it in the fridge for several days before freezing.

Reheating food

• It is safe to thaw purees in a microwave or saucepan as long as the food is heated all the way through until piping hot. Allow to cool down, and stir thoroughly before giving to your baby.

• Do not reheat food more than once, and do not save your baby's half-eaten food, as bacteria-carrying saliva from the spoon will have been introduced.

• Your baby's food should be given warm but not too hot, as a baby's mouth is more sensitive to heat than an adult's.

• If reheating in a microwave, heat until piping hot and allow to cool. This is to destroy any bacteria that might be present in the food.

• When reheating food in a microwave, stir thoroughly to get rid of any hot spots. Check the temperature before giving to your baby.

Food allergies

The greatest incidence of food allergy occurs in the first few years of life. However, there is no need to be unduly worried about it unless there is a family history of allergy or atopic disease, such as hay fever, asthma, or eczema. The incidence of food allergy in most babies is actually very small—about 6 percent.

The most common foods that carry the risk of allergic reaction in babies are:

• cow's milk and dairy products

• nuts and seeds

• eggs

• wheat-based products

• fish, especially shellfish

• berry and citrus fruits, which can trigger a reaction but rarely cause a true allergy

If one or both parents or a sibling has a history of food allergy or atopic disease, your baby will have an increased risk of developing an allergic disorder, and foods should only be introduced singly and under careful observation. It is best to take the following precautions:

• If possible, breast-feed exclusively for the first six months. If this is not possible, discuss with your doctor the option of using a "hypoallergenic" infant formula instead.
• When weaning, avoid the high-risk foods listed above until your baby is at least six months old. Instead start with foods that are unlikely to provoke an allergic reaction, such as baby rice, root vegetables, apples, and pears.
• New food groups should be introduced one at a time over 2 to 3 days. In that way, if there is a reaction, you will know what has caused it.
• If there is a family history of allergy to a particular food, avoid it until your child is at least six months old.
• If you suspect your child could be allergic to wheat or cow's milk, do not exclude key foods like these from your child's diet without first consulting a doctor.

> Although a lot of children grow out of their allergies by the age of three, some allergies—particularly a sensitivity to eggs, milk, fish, shellfish, or nuts—can last for life.

What is an allergic reaction?

An allergic reaction generally occurs when the immune system wrongly identifies a harmless substance as a threat and triggers the production of large amounts of antibodies in the blood, which can cause or contribute to various conditions such as eczema, urticaria (itchy red or white raised patches), hay fever, asthma, diarrhea, and even failure to thrive. If your child is found to be allergic to a basic food like wheat or cow's milk, you should seek expert advice on how to keep meals balanced.

Food intolerance

A food intolerance, sometimes referred to as a "false" food allergy, is a condition whereby the body is incapable of digesting certain foods properly. The condition is generally short-lived and not the same as a true food allergy, which involves the immune system. However, it can provoke the same symptoms, so if you suspect that your child is allergic to a common food like cow's milk, you should consult your pediatrician before changing the milk formula. It is quite possible that your baby's adverse reaction to it is only temporary.

How a food allergy is diagnosed

A food allergy can trigger a wide range of symptoms, from vomiting, itching, and swelling in the mouth, throat, and skin, to persistent diarrhea, abdominal pain, eczema, skin rashes, and wheezing. With so many symptoms that could have other causes, it is often hard to be sure that food is to blame, or to find out which food. Reactions may occur immediately after eating a specific food or may be delayed for hours or even days. If you are worried that your child might be allergic to a certain food, you should seek expert medical advice.

Now that solid foods tend to be introduced from six months—later than before—allergic reactions to foods in young infants is not seen as often as was previously the case. However, it is still babies under the age of eighteen months who are most likely to develop an allergy.

Many people blame food additives, but reactions to these are probably at least a hundred times less common than reactions to natural foods such as milk or wheat.

The only accurate way to diagnose a food allergy is to eliminate the suspected or most common allergens, wait for symptoms to cease, and, after a period of up to six weeks, reintroduce them one by one until the symptoms reappear. This type of "elimination" diet should be done only under medical supervision and with the help of a registered dietician. Other methods, such as electrode testing and kinesiology, do not provide an accurate means of diagnosing food allergies.

Allergy to cow's milk protein

This is the most commonly occurring food allergy and affects about 3 percent of children. An allergic reaction to infant formula or any dairy product can occur in a matter of minutes, or even after a few days. Symptoms can include cramps, diarrhea, vomiting, a skin rash, or breathing difficulties.

If your baby is sensitive to cow's milk–based infant formula, consult your doctor, who should recommend a specially designed hypoallergenic formula, available by prescription. This has quite a distinctive flavor, and whereas breast milk tastes sweet, this can be a little bitter. You may find that your baby may not be keen on this milk if you are still breast-feeding, but persevere; once you have stopped breast-feeding, she should get used to the taste.

Breast milk is the best milk for babies, but occasionally breast-feeding mothers may need to eliminate dairy foods from their own diets, as these can be transferred to their babies through breast milk. Only do this following the recommendation of your doctor, however.

All dairy products—such as cheese, yogurt, butter, ice cream, and chocolate—must be eliminated from the diet if your child has an allergy to cow's milk protein. In some less severe cases— for example, where cow's milk allergy causes eczema—small amounts of dairy products may be tolerated.

You should give your baby soy-based infant formula only if your GP or pediatrician advises you to. In almost all cases, breast milk or another type of formula will be a better choice. Soy-based infant milks are not recommended for babies under six months due to the high level of phytoestrogen, which could pose a risk to long-term reproductive health. It is probably best to avoid giving infant soy milk to your baby as a main drink for the first year. Also, bear in mind that children under two should not be given standard supermarket soy milk as their main drink—they need a special infant formula, as it provides more nutrients.

Because they weigh much less, babies take in a higher proportion of phytoestrogen when they drink soy-based infant formula compared with older children who eat some soy products as part of a mixed diet.

You can still use the recipes in this book if your baby has an allergy to cow's milk. Sweetened soy milk and soy margarine make good substitutes for ordinary cow's milk or butter when cooking for your baby. You could also use sunflower margarine, and many soy-based yogurts and desserts are available. Carob can be substituted for milk chocolate. However, some soy cheeses contain milk traces and therefore may be unsuitable.

If dairy products have to be avoided, it is important to introduce alternative sources of calcium. These can include milk-free cheeses, tofu, leafy green vegetables, dried fruit, seeds, bread, and fortified soy drinks.

Lactose intolerance

Lactose is the sugar present in milk. Lactose intolerance is the inability to digest this sugar because of a lack in the gut of a digestive enzyme known as lactase. It is not actually an allergy. The main symptoms are diarrhea, cramping, flatulence, and abdominal distension. Lactose intolerance can be hereditary—where the body simply does not produce sufficient amounts of lactase—or it can follow a period of gastroenteritis (infection in the gut). Following gastroenteritis, the sites where the enzyme lactase is produced may be damaged and therefore the lactose remains undigested, causing problems. In a few weeks to months, the enzyme begins to be produced once more and lactose is digested normally again.

Some children may benefit from a milk-free diet for a short period of time. You could give a hydrolyzed formula instead, following consultation with your doctor.

When buying food, you need to look out for items that have milk in the ingredients but under a different name—such as casein, caseinates, nonfat milk, and whey. Sometimes children who are lactose intolerant are able to tolerate small amounts of hard cheese (with lower levels of lactose) and yogurts (in which the lactose is digested by bacteria), but this depends very much on the individual child.

Peanut allergy

In the case of peanuts and peanut-based products—which can induce a severe allergic reaction, such as anaphylactic shock, that can be life threatening—it is best to err on the side of caution. In families with a history of any kind of food allergy, it is advisable to avoid all products containing peanuts until the child is three years old and then seek medical advice before introducing them into the diet. Vegetable oils that may contain peanut oil aren't a problem, as the oil is refined, thereby removing any traces of peanut protein. However, peanut butter and finely ground nuts can be introduced from six months, provided there is no family history of allergy. Whole nuts should not be given to children under the age of five because of the risk of choking.

Eggs

It is usually the protein in egg white that babies are allergic to. Your baby's mouth may swell quickly after being touched by egg, and hives (itchy red or whitish raised patches) are also a common reaction. It is amazing how many foods contain eggs—unless bakery products are labeled with the ingredients, it is always safer to assume that they contain eggs. Egg products may also be listed as albumen, lecithin E322, ovoglobulin, globulin, ovalblumen, ovomucin, or vitellin. You can buy egg alternatives in the supermarket.

Gluten intolerance

Gluten is found in wheat and other cereals such as rye and barley, and is therefore present in basic foods like bread, pasta, breakfast cereals, cake, and cookies. Celiac disease, a permanent sensitivity to gluten, is a serious medical condition. If there is a family history of celiac disease, there is an increased risk that your child will also suffer from it. Symptoms of celiac disease in your child may include loss of appetite, poor growth, swollen abdomen, and pale, frothy, and smelly stools. The disease is diagnosed medically by a blood test and can be confirmed by actually looking at the gut wall using endoscopy. This needs to be done before wheat is excluded from the diet, otherwise the test may give a false result.

As previously stated, foods containing gluten should not be introduced into any baby's diet before six months. Cereals introduced between 4 and 6 months should be gluten free, such as rice or corn. Baby rice is the safest at first. Thereafter, substitute rice, rice noodles, or buckwheat spaghetti for wheat pasta, and rice- or corn-based cereals for wheat-based varieties at breakfast. Gluten-free bread, flour, pasta, and cakes are also available.

Research shows that most celiacs can eat moderate portions of oats (for example, a bowl of oatmeal). Corn flour or white, brown, or ground rice or potato flour can be used instead of wheat flour.

Food additives and colorings

Some widely used food additives, like the food coloring tartrazine, have been associated with allergic reactions in a small minority of children. Some links have also been reported between hyperactivity and additives in the diet. There is some evidence that in a small minority additives, such as artificial flavorings and colorings, or natural foods such as milk or wheat, may change behavior. However, as stated above, this is true of only a very small minority—a much lower incidence than is perceived by parents.

Check the label on dried apricots to make sure they have not been treated with sulfur dioxide. This substance can trigger an asthma attack in a very small number of susceptible babies.

• For information on food allergies, contact the Food Allergy & Anaphylaxis Network, www.foodallergy.org, or the National Institutes of Health, www.nim.nih.gov/medlineplus/foodallergy.html
• For information on celiac disease, contact the Celiac Disease Foundation, www.celiac.org
• For information on eczema, contact the National Eczema Society, www.eczema.org
• For information on lactose intolerance, visit http://digestive.niddk.nih.gov/ddiseases/pubs/lactoseintolerance/

Eczema

Eczema is a complicated subject, and children with eczema should always be examined by their GP. Eczema is often not due to food but to other factors such as laundry detergents, soaps, or grass or other pollens in the air. If there is a history of eczema in the family, then breast-feeding may help delay the onset of the condition. The foods most commonly implicated in food allergies that may present as eczema are cow's milk, nuts, wheat, eggs, and shellfish.

Weaning preterm babies

If your baby was born prematurely, weaning times can vary. Babies born before thirty-seven weeks are considered preterm and have a greater need for certain nutrients like iron and zinc because these start to be stored in your baby's body in the last months of pregnancy.

A lot of preterm babies will be ready for solid food before six months' "corrected" age (i.e., the age of a child calculated from his expected date of delivery). It is advised that preterm babies be introduced to solids at some point between four and seven months' "uncorrected" age (i.e., the age of a child calculated from his actual, rather than expected, date of delivery).

There are no particular signs that a baby might give to show that he is ready to start weaning, and this should be discussed with your pediatrician and other health professionals involved in your baby's feeding to ensure that you do not start too early. On the other hand, it seems that making sure lumpy food is not introduced too late may help prevent some feeding difficulties. It has been suggested that babies should be eating food consisting of some soft lumps at least by nine months' uncorrected age. Allowing your baby to have finger foods as soon as he can cope with them will probably also encourage him to accept different foods more readily, as well as helping in the development of hand-eye coordination.

Moderately premature babies are able to be breast-fed, but despite scientific evidence showing that nursing offers clear benefits to "preemies," doctors and nurses do not always encourage it. This is because they are concerned with strictly controlling the amount of milk the baby takes. As a result, most babies in neonatal intensive care are given either pumped breast milk or formula. For mothers who pump milk while their babies are in the hospital, this has significant nutritional benefits and helps to create immunities; however, this can be pretty hard work. Bear in mind that most of breast milk's physiological benefits in terms of immunogenic protection are achieved within the first few months. If breast milk is unavailable, premature babies are given a special infant formula that contains more calories, protein, vitamins, and minerals than standard formula milk. Preterm babies tend to be in a state of "catch up" in terms of growth, and they often need larger volumes of milk and require feeding more frequently than full-term babies.

Care needs to be taken when weaning preterm babies to ensure that foods are not too low in energy—it is no good filling your baby up with fruit and vegetable purees, thereby displacing the nutrients that milk provides. Foods like eggs, cheese, yogurt, and avocado are ideal nutrient-dense foods for the second stage of weaning, as are potato- or sweet-potato-based purees made with the special formula or breast milk or with a little added butter or olive oil. Baby rice (which is fortified with iron) mixed with the special formula or breast milk is good for breakfast, but try adding some fruit puree to alter the flavor. Contrary to popular belief, babies don't always prefer food that tastes bland. You also need to ensure that you include foods that provide good sources of protein and iron. Introduce meat at around six months and, a little later, fish. If you don't want to give your baby meat or fish, small amounts of pureed beans, peas, or lentils make a good alternative. Offer a wide variety of foods, to ensure a good nutritional balance and to discourage your baby from being a fussy eater later on.

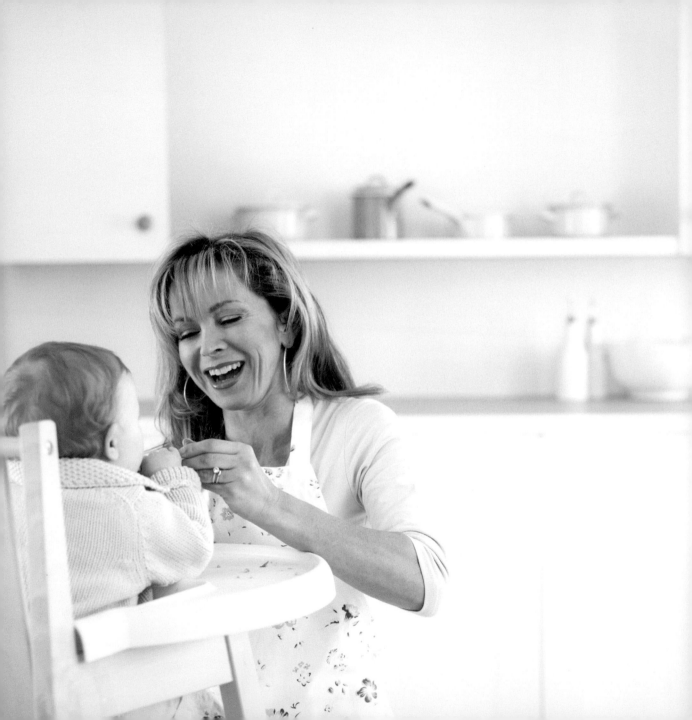

First-stage weaning: 6 months

Weaning your baby from milk to solids is an important and exciting milestone for both of you, and it's a big step forward for your baby, as it opens up a whole new world of taste.

There is nothing better for your baby than freshly prepared food, and my puree recipes are quick and easy to make. Most are suitable for freezing, so that you don't have to cook them from scratch every day. By making baby food yourself, you can be sure of using only the best-quality ingredients, and homemade purees taste so much better than jars of baby food, which often have a shelf life of up to two years.

Keep to the main guidelines and then follow your instincts because no two babies are the same, and Mom usually knows best.

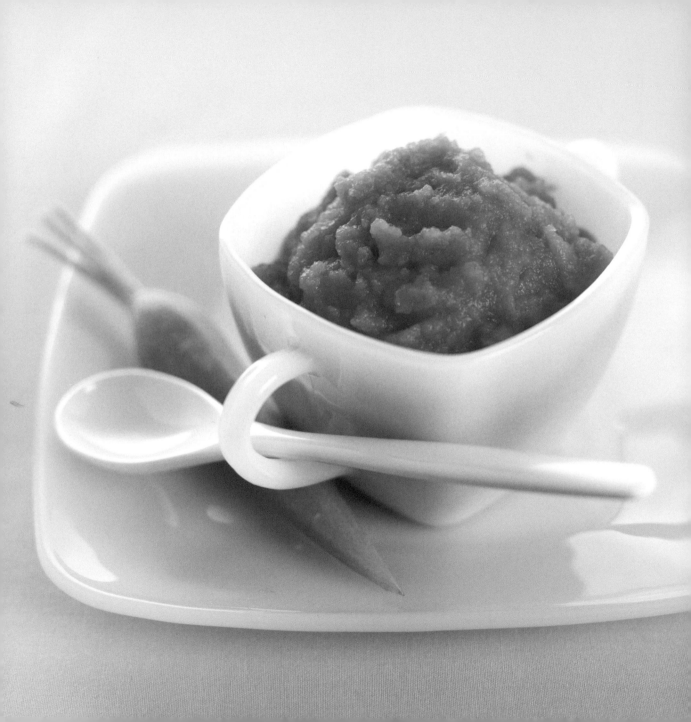

First vegetable puree

4 to 6 medium carrots (12 ounces), peeled and chopped

Put the carrots in a steamer set over boiling water and cook for 15 to 20 minutes or until tender. Alternatively, put the carrots in a saucepan and add just enough boiling water to cover. Cover and simmer for 15 to 20 minutes or until soft.

Drain the carrots and place in a blender, adding some of the water from the bottom of the steamer or some of the cooking liquid, then puree until very smooth. The amount of liquid you add really depends on your baby; you may need to add a little more if he finds the puree difficult to swallow. Spoon some of the puree into your baby's bowl and serve lukewarm.

Food fact: Interestingly, carrots are more nutritious when cooked with a little fat, such as a pat of unsalted butter, as the beta-carotene they contain is absorbed more readily.

Carrots make excellent weaning food, as babies like their naturally sweet taste.

TOP TIP
It isn't a good idea to delay introducing solids any later than six months. Your baby needs to learn how to chew and swallow food, and learning to chew also encourages the development of the muscles that are essential for speech.

Baby rice should be the first cereal you introduce because it does not contain gluten, a protein that is found in cereals like wheat, barley, and rye, and that can cause food allergy if introduced before six months.

TOP TIP
Allow plenty of time for feeding when first introducing solids. Go at your baby's pace. While sucking is a natural reflex, your baby needs to learn to move solid food from the front of the tongue to the back, in order to swallow it.

Creamy vegetable or fruit puree

1 tablespoon baby rice cereal
3 tablespoons your baby's usual milk
¼ cup vegetable or fruit puree
    (see page 23 or 25)

Mix the baby rice and milk together according to the instructions on the package and stir into the vegetable or fruit puree.

6 MONTHS

MAKES 6 PORTIONS

COOKING TIME: 4–8 MINUTES

SUITABLE FOR FREEZING

Apples make an easily digested introduction to fruit.

First fruit puree

2 medium apples or pears, peeled, cored, and chopped
2 tablespoons water or unsweetened apple juice
  (optional)

Put the chopped fruit into a heavy-bottomed saucepan and, if using apples, add the water or apple juice; ripe pears will not need any extra liquid. Cover and cook over low heat until tender (6 to 8 minutes for apples and about 4 minutes for pears). Blend the fruit to a puree. Spoon a little into your baby's bowl and serve lukewarm.

Food fact: Apples and pears contain pectin, which can slow things down if your baby has loose stools. Pectin is a soluble fiber that also helps to stimulate bacteria in the gut and helps a baby's bowels to start processing solids efficiently.

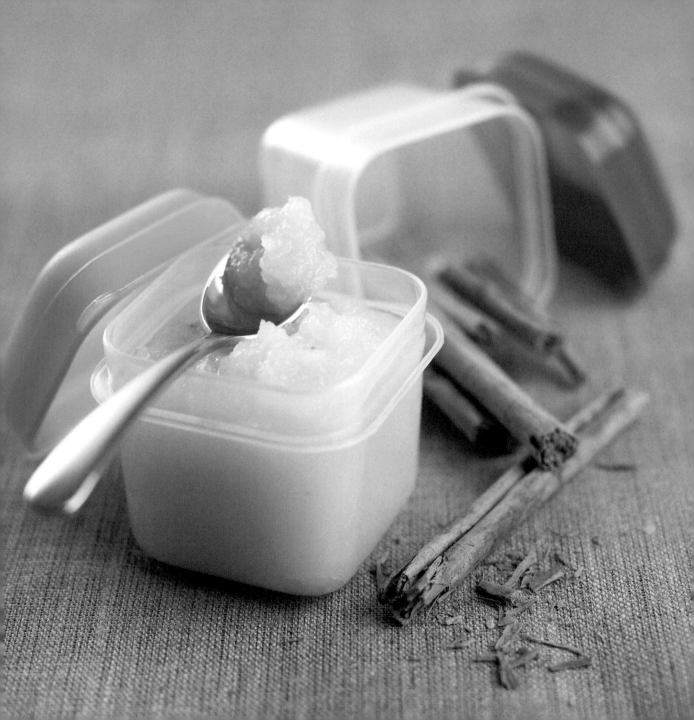

⊙ 6 MONTHS

🥄 MAKES 4 PORTIONS

🕐 COOKING TIME: 6–8 MINUTES

❄ SUITABLE FOR FREEZING

Apple and pear with cinnamon

2 medium apples, peeled, cored, and chopped
2 medium pears, peeled, cored, and chopped
¼ cup unsweetened apple juice or water
Generous pinch of ground cinnamon (optional)

Put the fruit into a saucepan together with the apple juice or water and cinnamon (if using), cover, and cook over low heat for 6 minutes or until tender. Blend the fruit to a smooth puree.

Apple and pear puree is an ideal first food, being easy to digest and unlikely to cause allergies. Choose sweet apples like Golden Delicious or Royal Gala. Some varieties, such as Granny Smith, may have too tart a flavor for your baby.

TOP TIP
Weaning spoons should be sterilized for the first six months. However, once your baby is crawling around and testing objects in her mouth, there is little point in sterilizing anything other than bottles and nipples. Your baby's bowls can be washed in the dishwasher or in very hot water.

6 MONTHS

MAKES 3 PORTIONS

COOKING TIME: 12 MINUTES

SUITABLE FOR FREEZING

Broccoli is best steamed or microwaved, as boiling halves its vitamin C content. If your baby isn't keen on the flavor, mix it with a sweet-tasting vegetable like sweet potato, rutabaga, butternut squash, or pumpkin. As a variation on this recipe, try sweet potato and peas or sweet potato and spinach.

Sweet potato and broccoli

1 medium sweet potato (8 ounces), peeled and chopped
¾ cup broccoli florets
1 tablespoon unsalted butter
1 to 2 tablespoons your baby's usual milk

Steam the sweet potato and broccoli until tender (the sweet potato for about 12 minutes; broccoli for 6 to 7 minutes). Alternatively, place the sweet potato in a saucepan, cover with water, and boil for 4 minutes, then add the broccoli and continue to boil for 6 to 7 minutes. Puree together with the butter and milk.

6 MONTHS

MAKES 4 PORTIONS

COOKING TIME:
12 MINUTES/1 ¹/₂ HOURS

SUITABLE FOR FREEZING

Butternut squash makes a good combination with vegetables like peas or broccoli and also goes well with fruits like apple or pear.

Butternut squash

1 medium butternut squash (1 pound), peeled,
*   cut in half, and seeded*
1 tablespoon unsalted butter (optional)
2 tablespoons orange juice (optional)

Chop the butternut squash into pieces and steam or boil for about 12 minutes, then puree. Alternatively, brush each half with melted butter and spoon 1 tablespoon orange juice into each cavity. Cover with foil and bake in a preheated oven at 350°F for 1½ hours or until tender, then blend to a puree.

Food fact: Butternut squash is easily digested, rarely causes allergies, and provides a good source of beta-carotene. Just 1 cup provides an adult with approximately 300 percent of the vitamin A (beta-carotene) needed for a whole day.

Trio of root vegetables

1 medium sweet potato (8 ounces), peeled and chopped
2 to 3 medium carrots, peeled and chopped
1 medium parsnip (4 ounces), peeled and chopped

Steam the vegetables for about 20 minutes or until tender. Blend to a puree, adding a little of the boiled water from the bottom of the steamer, or some of your baby's usual milk, to make the right consistency for him.

If you don't have a steamer, put the vegetables into a saucepan and barely cover with boiling water. Cover the pan and cook over medium heat for about 20 minutes or until tender. Drain the vegetables and blend to a puree using a little of the cooking liquid or some of your baby's usual milk.

Food fact: Orange-fleshed sweet potato is a good source of vitamin C and beta-carotene, and is richer in nutrients than ordinary potatoes.

6 MONTHS

MAKES 6 PORTIONS

COOKING TIME: 20 MINUTES

SUITABLE FOR FREEZING

Root vegetables have a naturally sweet taste, puree to a smooth consistency, and are unlikely to cause allergies, so they make a good first food. You could substitute sweet potato with another vegetable like rutabaga or pumpkin.

Raw fruits are more nutritious than cooked, since no nutrients are lost. You can combine two different fruits, as in Avocado or Papaya and Banana (see opposite).

No-cook baby food

Avocado

Cut a small avocado in half, remove the pit, scoop out the flesh, and mash together with a little of your baby's usual milk.

Food fact: Avocados are sometimes thought of as a vegetable, but they are actually a fruit and contain more nutrients than any other type of fruit. They are a great source of the free-radical-fighting antioxidant vitamin E, which also boosts the immune system. In addition, they are rich in monounsaturated fat, the "good" type of fat that helps prevent heart disease. The high calorie content of avocados makes them an ideal food for growing babies.

Banana

Mash a small banana with a fork. During the first stages of weaning, add a little of your baby's usual milk, if necessary, to thin down the consistency and provide a familiar taste.

Food fact: Bananas are full of slow-release sugars that provide sustained energy. They are also good for the treatment of both diarrhea and constipation. Make sure you choose ripe bananas; they will have brown spots on the skin.

Papaya

Cut a small papaya in half, peel, remove the black seeds, and puree or mash the flesh of one half until smooth.

Food fact: Papaya contains papain, an enzyme that breaks down protein and so boosts the digestion, as well as improving indigestion. It is rich in vitamin C and beta-carotene. A 3-ounce portion of papaya will provide a young child's daily requirement of vitamin C. Papaya is also high in soluble fiber, which is important for normal bowel function.

Avocado or papaya and banana

½ small avocado or ½ small papaya
½ small banana
1 to 2 tablespoons your baby's usual milk

Mash the avocado or papaya together with the banana and the milk. If using papaya, the milk is optional.

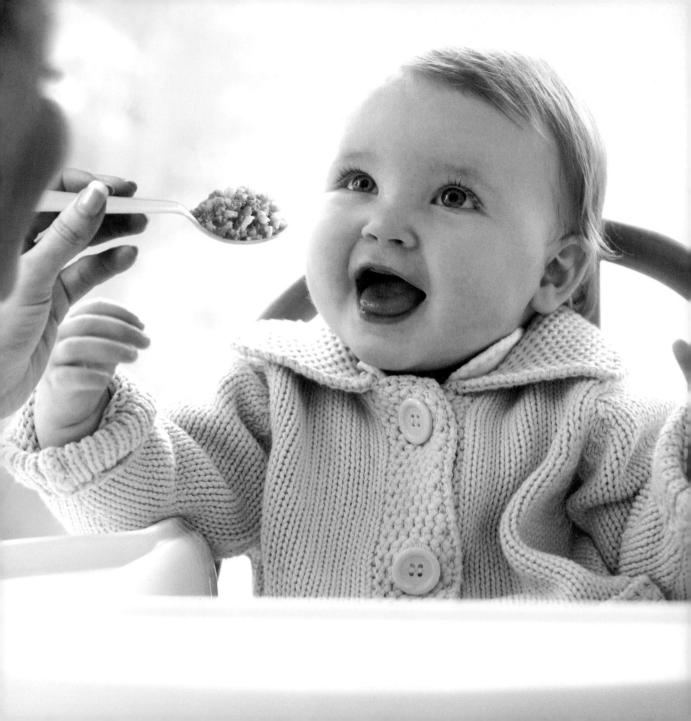

After first tastes: 6 to 7 months

Try to wean your baby onto as wide a range of foods as possible.
After first tastes are accepted, you can pretty well introduce all fruits
and vegetables. However, take care with citrus, pineapple, berries, and
kiwifruit, as these may upset the stomachs of some susceptible babies.

   As well as fruit and vegetable purees, make sure you include foods
that are both nutritious and quite high in calories, such as full-fat
yogurt or cheese, as babies need these to fuel their rapid growth.

   In addition, it is important to include foods rich in iron, such as
red meat, as iron deficiency is the most common nutritional deficiency
in babies. As we saw in the Introduction, babies are born with an iron
store that lasts for about six months, and a baby's iron requirements
are particularly high between the ages of six months and two years.
This is a critical time for the growth of the brain, and a lack of iron
in the diet can lead to impaired mental development.

6–7 MONTHS

SEE INDIVIDUAL RECIPES
FOR PORTIONS

COOKING TIMES: SEE
INDIVIDUAL RECIPES

SUITABLE FOR FREEZING

Simple vegetable purees

Broccoli or cauliflower

Place about ½ pound small broccoli or cauliflower florets in a steamer and cook for about 10 minutes or until tender. Alternatively, put in a pan with enough water to cover, bring to a boil, cover, and simmer for about 6 minutes. Drain and blend to a puree. This works well mixed with potato, carrot, or sweet potato. It makes 6 portions.

Corn on the cob

Remove the outer husk and silk from the corn on the cob and rinse the cob well. Cover with boiling water and cook over medium heat for 10 minutes. Strain and then remove the kernels of corn using a sharp knife. Puree in a food mill. Alternatively, cook 1 cup frozen corn and then puree. This is good combined with carrot, leek, and potato, or chicken, leek, and potato. It makes 2 portions.

Zucchini

Place 3 small trimmed and sliced zucchini in a steamer and cook for about 10 minutes or until tender. Alternatively, put in a pan with enough water to cover, bring to a boil, cover, and simmer for about 6 minutes. Drain and blend to a puree. This makes a good combination with sweet potato, or leek, potato, and peas. It makes 8 portions.

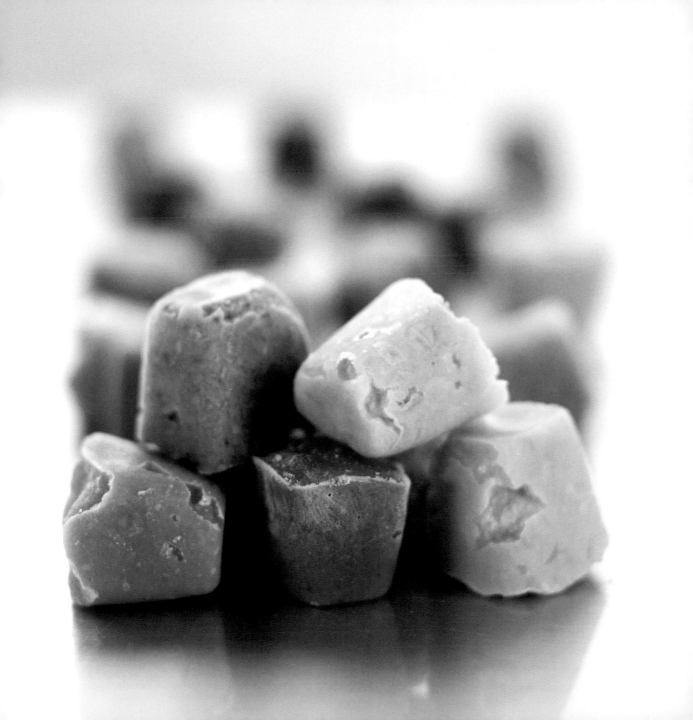

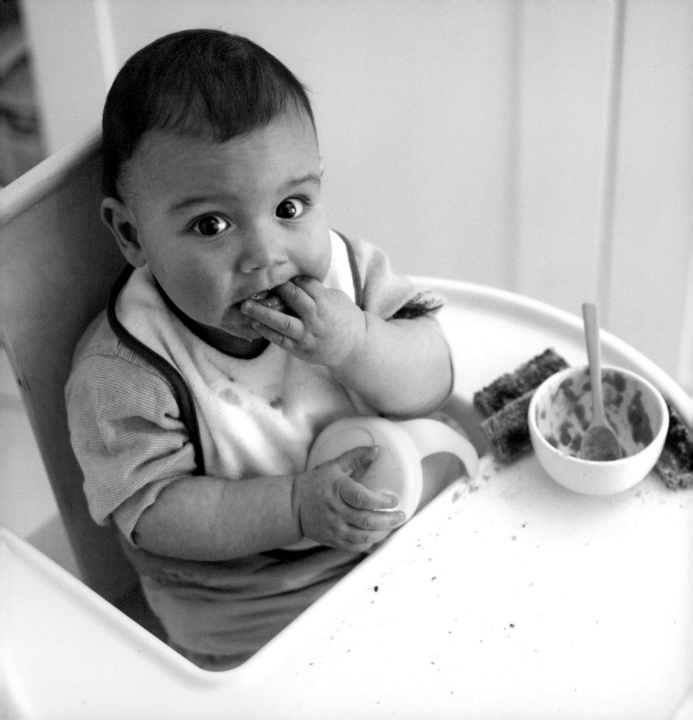

Peas

I tend to use frozen peas, as they are just as nutritious as the fresh variety. Cover 1½ cups peas with water, bring to a boil, cover, and simmer for 4 minutes or until tender. (If using fresh peas, cook them for about 15 minutes or until tender.) Drain, reserving some cooking liquid, then puree using a food mill. This puree works well combined with potato, carrot, or sweet potato. It makes 2 portions.

Spinach

Carefully wash 1 cup baby spinach leaves, removing the tough stems. Either steam the spinach or put in a saucepan and sprinkle with a little water. Cook for 3 to 4 minutes until the leaves are wilted. Gently press out any excess water, then puree in a blender. This works well combined with potato, sweet potato, or butternut squash. It makes 1 portion.

Sweet potato, rutabaga, or parsnip

Use a large sweet potato, a small rutabaga, or 2 parsnips. Peel and chop into chunks. Steam the vegetables for about 12 minutes or until tender. Alternatively, cover with boiling water and simmer, covered, for about 15 minutes or until tender. Drain, reserving the cooking liquid. Puree in a blender, adding some of the liquid if necessary. This makes 4 portions.

Tomato

Peel, seed, and roughly chop 2 medium tomatoes (see page 126). Melt a pat of unsalted butter in a heavy-bottomed saucepan and sauté the tomato until mushy. Puree in a blender. This is good combined with potato, cauliflower, or zucchini and a little grated cheese melted into the cooked tomatoes. It makes 1 portion.

Apricots can be quite sour, so taste them first and only give them to your baby if they are sweet. Mango, on the other hand, is naturally sweet and easy to digest, but do make sure you choose a ripe fruit. Most melons are also good, as they tend to be naturally sweet, and cantaloupes are very rich in vitamin A.

Simple fruit purees

Fresh apricot

Peel 2 large apricots in the same way as a peach or nectarine (see page 126), then puree using a handheld electric blender. This combines well with banana.

Food fact: Apricots are rich in beta-carotene and are a good source of iron and potassium. Dried apricots are particularly nutritious, as well as being rich in fiber. Make sure they have not been treated with sulfur dioxide to preserve the bright orange color and prevent fungus growth. This substance can trigger an asthma attack in susceptible babies.

Mango

Peel the fruit and slice down each side of the pit. Cut the flesh of half a mango into cubes and puree. This combines well with banana, strawberry, or yogurt.

Food fact: Mango is rich in vitamins A and C.

Melon

Remove the seeds from a small wedge of melon and cut the flesh away from the skin, discarding the greener flesh near the skin. Mash or blend to a puree of the desired consistency. This puree combines well with strawberries or banana.

Food fact: Cantaloupes are the most nutritious of all the melon varieties; they are rich in vitamin C and also provide beta-carotene and potassium.

Peach or nectarine

Peel a small, ripe peach or nectarine and chop the flesh (see page 126), then puree in a blender or mash. This puree works well combined with strawberries, banana, or blueberries.

Plum

Peel 2 large plums in the same way as a peach or nectarine (see page 126), then chop the flesh. Plums can be pureed uncooked if sufficiently soft and juicy, or you could steam them for a few minutes until tender. They are good mixed with baby rice, banana, or yogurt.

Dried fruit (apricot, peach, or prune)

Cover ½ cup fruit with water, bring to a boil, and simmer for about 5 minutes or until soft. Drain (remove pits from prunes if not pitted) and puree. Add a little of the cooking liquid to make a smooth puree. This can be combined with baby rice and milk or banana, pear, or apple puree.

Carrots are more nutritious when cooked, unlike many other vegetables. Cooking breaks open the plant cells so that antioxidants and other nutrients can be absorbed more easily by our bodies. It is better to steam rutabagas rather than boil them, as the vitamin C they contain is water soluble and much of it would be lost in the cooking water.

This would also be good with sweet potato or butternut squash instead of the rutabaga.

Rutabaga, carrot, and peas

1 medium rutabaga (8 ounces), peeled and chopped
3 medium carrots, peeled and chopped
½ cup frozen peas

Put the chopped rutabaga and carrots into a steamer and cook for 15 minutes. Alternatively, cover with water in a pan, bring to a boil, cover, and simmer for about 15 minutes. Add the frozen peas and continue to cook for another 5 minutes.

Puree in a blender with as much of the liquid from the bottom of the steamer (or pan) as needed to achieve a smooth consistency. For very young babies, you could puree this in a food mill to get rid of the skins from the peas.

Food facts: Just one large carrot provides the recommended daily intake of vitamin A for an adult. The darker a carrot is, the more vitamin A it contains, so choose older carrots over baby carrots. Carrots are particularly susceptible to chemicals in the soil, so it's a good idea to choose organic carrots. Rutabagas provide a good source of vitamin C.

See-in-the-dark puree

6–7 MONTHS

MAKES 6 PORTIONS

COOKING TIME: 24 MINUTES

SUITABLE FOR FREEZING

1 small onion, sliced
2 tablespoons unsalted butter
1 pound carrots, peeled and chopped
1½ cups Vegetable or Chicken Stock
    (see pages 124 and 125)
¼ cup orange juice

Sauté the onion in the butter until softened. Add the carrots and sauté for 3 to 4 minutes. Pour in the stock, bring to a boil, then reduce the heat and simmer for about 20 minutes or until the carrots are tender. Add the orange juice and puree in a blender.

Food fact: Carrots do improve night vision. They are an excellent source of beta-carotene, the plant form of vitamin A, and one of the first symptoms of vitamin A deficiency is night blindness.

Instead of potato, you could substitute sweet potato, butternut squash, or pumpkin in this recipe.

Potato, summer squash, and peas

½ cup finely chopped onion
1 tablespoon unsalted butter
1 small summer squash, trimmed and thinly sliced
2 small potatoes (6 ounces), peeled and chopped
½ cup Vegetable or Chicken Stock
    (see pages 124 and 125)
¼ cup frozen peas

Sauté the onion in the butter for about 3 minutes or until softened. Add the squash and sauté for 1 minute. Add the potatoes, pour in the stock, then cover and simmer for 12 minutes. Add the frozen peas, bring to a boil, then reduce the heat and continue to cook for 3 minutes. Puree in a blender.

Food fact: All the yellow-fleshed squashes are good sources of beta-carotene, but in zucchini this vitamin is present in any significant amount only in the skin, so they are best cooked and eaten with the skin on.

Cinderella's pumpkin

6–7 MONTHS

MAKES 3–4 PORTIONS

COOKING TIME: 32 MINUTES

SUITABLE FOR FREEZING

1 tablespoon unsalted butter
¼ cup washed and sliced white part of a leek
Half a small pumpkin or butternut squash, peeled
   and cut into cubes (about 1 cup)
½ cup Vegetable or Chicken Stock
   (see pages 124 and 125)

Melt the butter in a saucepan and sauté the leek
until soft and lightly golden. Add the pumpkin or
butternut squash and continue to cook for 2 minutes.
Pour in the stock, bring to a boil, and then simmer,
covered, for 30 minutes or until the pumpkin is tender.
Puree in a blender, or mash with a fork for older babies.

This was one of my youngest daughter's favorite combinations—and it tastes so good you could make it as a soup for the rest of the family. If you can't find pumpkin, try butternut squash instead.

As a meaty variation on this recipe, you could add 2½ ounces chopped chicken breast with the pumpkin or butternut squash. Simmer, covered, for 15 rather than 30 minutes.

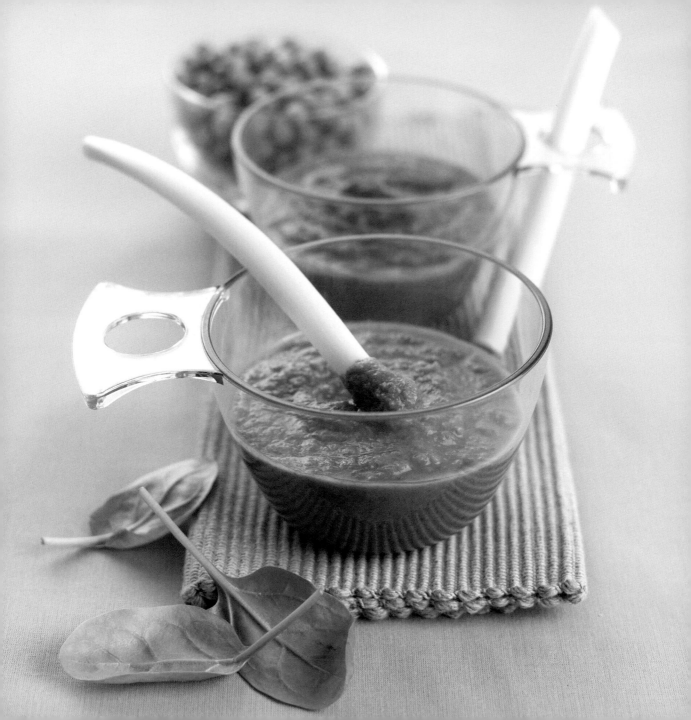

Sweet potato with spinach and peas

6–7 MONTHS

MAKES 5 PORTIONS

COOKING TIME: 14 MINUTES

SUITABLE FOR FREEZING

1 tablespoon unsalted butter
½ cup washed and sliced white part of a leek
1 large sweet potato (12 ounces), peeled and chopped
½ cup frozen peas
¾ cup fresh baby spinach (3 ounces), washed
*   and tough stems removed*

Melt the butter in a saucepan and sauté the leek for 2 to 3 minutes or until softened, then add the sweet potato. Pour in 1 cup water, bring to a boil, then cover and simmer for 7 to 8 minutes. Add the peas and spinach and cook for 3 minutes. Puree the vegetables in a blender to make a smooth consistency for your baby, adding a little of the cooking liquid if necessary.

Food fact: Frozen vegetables like peas can be just as nutritious as fresh, since they are frozen within hours of being picked, thus locking in vital nutrients. Once cooked, they can be refrozen.

Combining spinach with a sweet-tasting vegetable like sweet potato is a good way to introduce it to your baby. You can also make this recipe with broccoli instead of spinach.

For young babies it is best to puree corn through a food mill, as it will be easier to digest and have a smoother texture.

TOP TIP
Water is the best alternative drink to milk—ideally boiled, cooled tap water. Fully breast-fed babies don't need any water until they start eating solid food.

Potato, carrot, and corn

2 tablespoons unsalted butter
½ cup chopped onion
2 medium carrots, peeled and chopped
2 medium potatoes (8 ounces), peeled and chopped
1 cup Vegetable Stock (see page 124) or water
⅓ cup canned or frozen corn kernels
1 to 2 tablespoons milk

Melt the butter in a pan and sauté the onion for 1 minute. Add the carrots and sauté for 5 minutes. Add the potatoes, cover with the stock or water, and cook over medium heat for 15 minutes. Add the corn and continue to cook for 5 minutes. Puree through a food mill and stir in the milk to make the right consistency for your baby.

Food fact: Corn is a good source of beta-carotene and fiber.

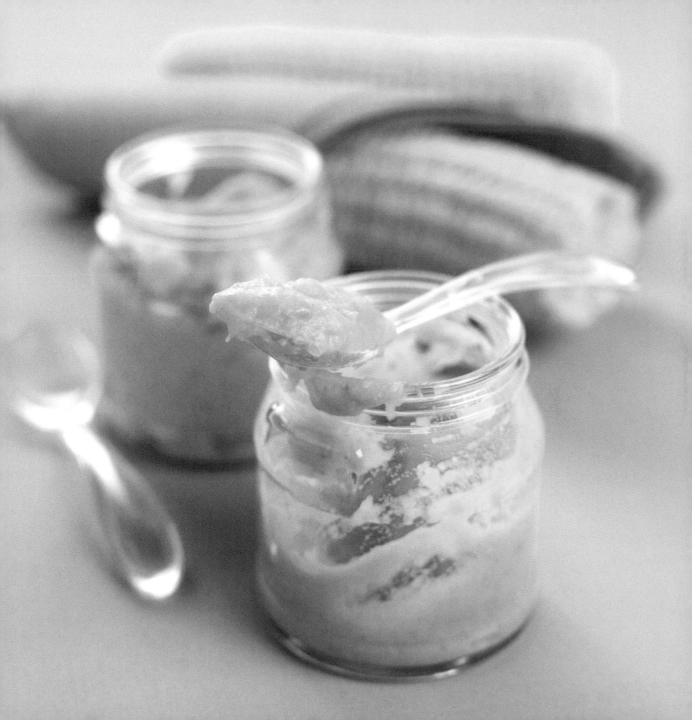

6–7 MONTHS

MAKES 4 PORTIONS

COOKING TIME: 23 MINUTES

SUITABLE FOR FREEZING

This tasty combination of fish and vegetables in a mild cheese sauce is very popular with babies.

TOP TIP
If your child has an allergy or intolerance, make sure you inform everyone who looks after your child.

Fillet of fish with cheese sauce and vegetables

1 tablespoon unsalted butter
½ cup washed and sliced white part of a leek
2 medium carrots, peeled and chopped
1 cup boiling water
½ cup frozen peas
5 ounces flounder or haddock fillet, skinned
½ cup milk
3 black peppercorns
1 bay leaf
Sprig of parsley

Cheese sauce
1 tablespoon unsalted butter
1 tablespoon all-purpose flour
½ cup grated Cheddar cheese

Melt the butter in a saucepan, add the leek, and sauté for 2 to 3 minutes. Add the carrots, cover with the boiling water, and cook for 15 minutes. Add the peas and cook for 5 minutes more, or until the vegetables are tender.

Meanwhile, put the fish in a pan with the milk, peppercorns, bay leaf, and parsley. Simmer for 3 to 4 minutes or until the fish is cooked. Flake the fish and set aside, reserving the cooking liquid. Discard the flavorings.

Make the cheese sauce (see page 126 for recipe), using the cooking liquid instead of milk.

Drain the vegetables and mix with the flaked fish and cheese sauce. Blend to a puree of the desired consistency for a young baby. Provided the vegetables are tender, this can be mashed for a younger baby or chopped for one who is beginning to chew.

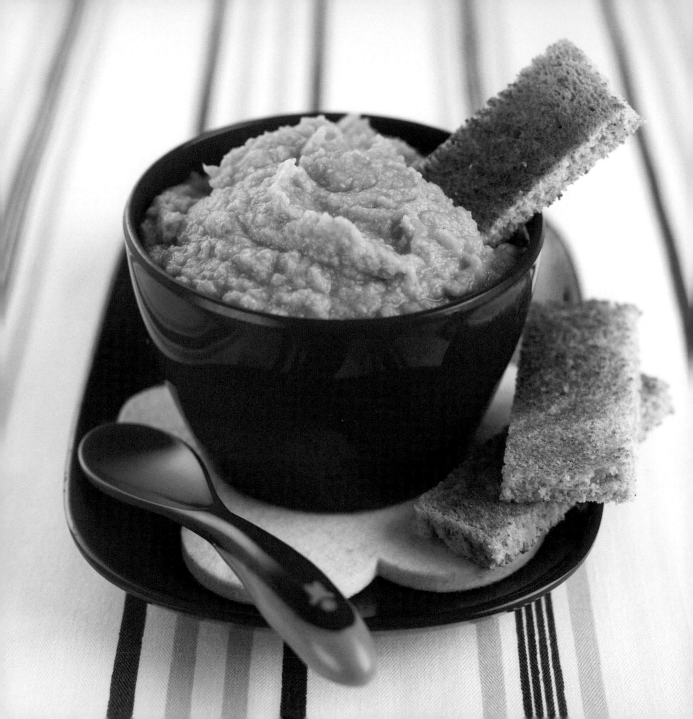

6–7 MONTHS

MAKES 4 PORTIONS

COOKING TIME: 20 MINUTES

SUITABLE FOR FREEZING

Chicken with sweet potato and apple

Apple and chicken make a delicious combination. Mixing it with sweet potato gives a smoother texture.

1 tablespoon unsalted butter
¼ cup chopped onion
4 ounces boneless, skinless chicken breast, chopped
1 large sweet potato (12 ounces), peeled and chopped
½ apple, peeled, cored, and chopped
1 cup Chicken Stock (see page 125)

Heat the butter in a saucepan, add the onion, and sauté for 2 to 3 minutes. Add the chicken and sauté for a couple of minutes until it turns opaque. Add the sweet potato and apple and pour in the stock. Bring to a boil, then cover and simmer for 15 minutes. Puree to the desired consistency.

Food fact: Chicken is an ideal "growth" food, as it is packed with protein and vitamin B_{12}, which is not found in plants.

Some purees are particularly easy to prepare, as they use ingredients that don't need to be cooked. Following are some delicious—and very nutritious—combinations for you to try. They are equally suitable for breakfast or dessert and can also be mixed with baby rice. Do make sure that the fruit is sweet and ripe by tasting it first yourself. For the purees with yogurt, always choose the whole-milk, unsweetened, natural, "live" variety for babies. Fresh peach and dried apricot also go well with yogurt.

Instant no-cook purees

Bananas (the base for most of these purees) are a great first food, as they are quick to prepare, easy to digest, and unlikely to cause an allergic reaction. In addition, they make perfect portable baby food, as they come in their own easy-to-peel "packaging."

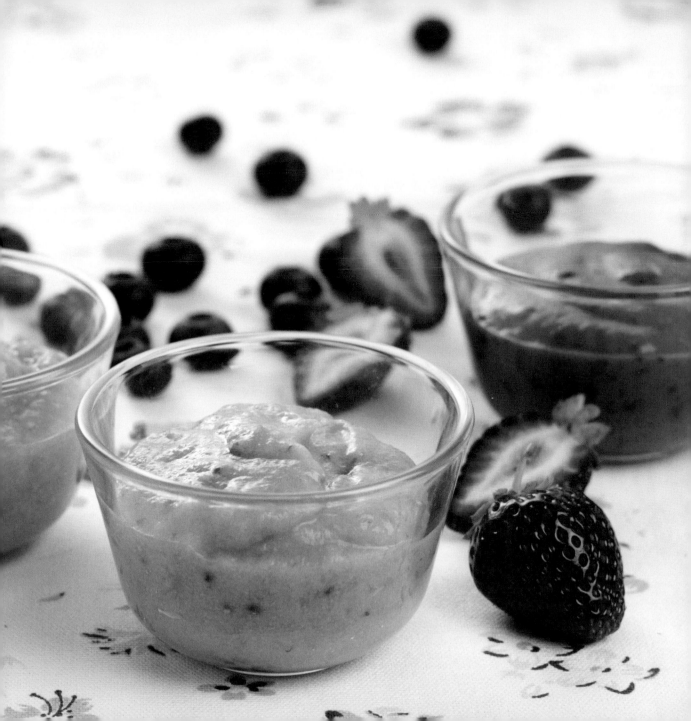

Banana and blueberry

¼ cup blueberries
1 small banana, sliced

Put the blueberries into a saucepan together with 1 tablespoon water, and cook for about 2 minutes or until the fruit just starts to burst open. Using a handheld electric blender, whiz the blueberries and banana together until smooth.

Banana and mango or papaya

1 small banana
1 small mango, peeled and pitted,
   or papaya, peeled and seeded

Slice the fruit and blend together.

Banana, peach, and strawberry

1 small banana, sliced
1 peach, peeled and pitted (see page 126)
2 strawberries, hulled and quartered

Blend the fruit together.

Banana with apple

1 small banana, sliced
2 to 3 tablespoons apple puree (see page 25)

Simply mash the banana together with the apple puree.

Cantaloupe and strawberry

½ cantaloupe , peeled,
   seeded, and chopped
3 strawberries, hulled and quartered
1 to 2 tablespoons baby rice cereal

Blend the fruit together and stir in the baby rice to thicken the puree.

Banana, avocado, and yogurt
½ small banana, sliced
½ small avocado
1 to 2 tablespoons yogurt

Mash or puree the banana together with the avocado, and stir in the yogurt.

Mango and yogurt
½ small mango, peeled and chopped
3 to 4 tablespoons mild, full-fat yogurt

Puree the mango using a handheld electric blender and mix together with the yogurt. This makes 2 portions.

Banana and pear
1 small banana, sliced
½ pear, peeled, cored, and chopped

Mash or puree the banana together with the pear.

Note: Purees of banana are best served at once, otherwise they discolor. Look for little brown spots on the banana skin to make sure it is really ripe.

Banana with tofu
1 small banana
¼ cup silken tofu

Mash the banana and mix together with the tofu. You could also mix tofu with other fruits like mango or peaches.

Food fact: Most vegetarians will know the health benefits of tofu, which is made from soybean curd. It makes an excellent high-protein alternative to meat and is rich in many nutrients, including iron, potassium, and calcium.

This is a delicious puree to make when sweet, ripe peaches are in season. Their natural sweetness makes them a favorite with little ones.

TOP TIP
It's best not to put anything into a bottle apart from milk or water. Comfort sucking on sweet drinks is the main cause of tooth decay in young children. It is a good idea to start using a lidded cup with a spout from the age of 6 to 7 months and eventually move on to an open cup.

Peach and banana

1 peach, peeled, pitted, and cut into pieces
(see page 126)
1 small banana, sliced
1½ teaspoons apple juice
A little baby rice cereal (optional)

Put the peach and banana into a small pan together with the apple juice, cover, and simmer for 2 to 3 minutes, then puree in a blender. If the puree is too runny, stir in a little baby rice.

Food fact: Peaches are a good source of vitamin C and easy to digest. Orange peaches are rich in immune-boosting vitamin C and beta-carotene, which will help your baby ward off illness.

Apple, strawberry, and peach

6–7 MONTHS

MAKES 4 PORTIONS

COOKING TIME: 5 MINUTES

SUITABLE FOR FREEZING

1 large apple, peeled, cored, and chopped
⅓ cup hulled and quartered strawberries
1 large peach, peeled, pitted, and chopped
   (see page 126)
1 tablespoon baby rice cereal

Put the fruit into a saucepan, cover, and cook over low heat for about 5 minutes. Puree in a blender and stir in the baby rice.

Food fact: Strawberries contain more vitamin C than other berry fruits and can help strengthen your child's immune defenses. Strawberries also contain ellagic acid, believed to help prevent cancer. Some babies with sensitive skin or eczema can have a reaction to eating berry fruits. Watch out for soreness around the mouth or irritation to the skin.

You could finely crush a baby zwieback and stir that into the fruit puree instead of the baby rice.

Also try strawberry and pear puree. Peel, core, and chop 2 ripe pears and place in a pan with ¼ cup hulled and quartered strawberries. Cook for 3 to 4 minutes. Puree in a blender and stir in 2 tablespoons baby rice to thicken.

This is an ideal puree for introducing young babies to chicken.

Easy one-pot chicken

½ cup washed and sliced white part of a leek
1 tablespoon unsalted butter
4 ounces boneless, skinless chicken breast,
*   cut into chunks*
1 medium carrot, peeled and sliced
1 large sweet potato (10 to 12 ounces),
*   peeled and chopped*
1¼ cups Chicken Stock (see page 125)

Sauté the leek in the butter until softened. Add the chicken to the pan and sauté for 3 to 4 minutes. Add the vegetables, pour in the stock, bring to a boil, and simmer, covered, for about 30 minutes or until the chicken is cooked through and the vegetables are tender. Puree in a blender to the desired consistency.

Peach, pear, and blueberry

1 juicy peach, peeled, pitted, and chopped
  (see page 126)
1 medium pear, peeled, cored, and chopped
½ cup blueberries
2 to 3 tablespoons baby rice cereal

Put the fruit into a small saucepan, cover, and cook over low heat for 3 to 4 minutes, stirring occasionally. Puree in a blender and stir in the baby rice while still hot.

Food fact: Blueberries are a good source of vitamin C and also contain beta-carotene. They have the highest antioxidant content of all fruits, mainly because of the blue pigment, anthocyanin, in their skin.

Soft fruits such as these tend to produce a runny fruit puree—adding baby rice is a good way to thicken the texture.

TOP TIP

Fruit juices are a good source of vitamin C, but bear in mind that giving your baby juices and other drinks will reduce his appetite for milk. Fruit juice is acidic and also contains natural sugars, which can cause tooth decay. It is best not to give your baby fruit juice before he is six months old, as some babies can have an adverse reaction to citrus fruit. All fruit juices should be diluted in the proportion of five parts water to one part juice.

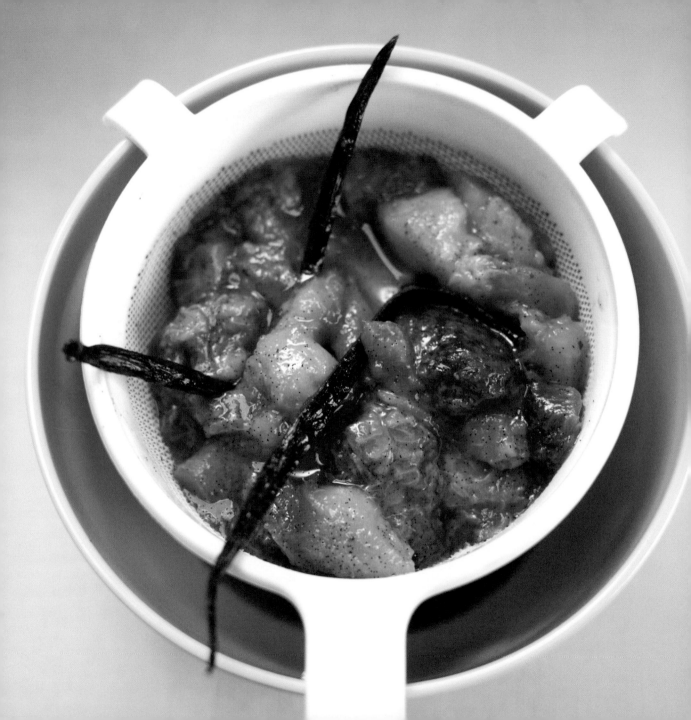

Apricot, apple, pear, and vanilla

3 ounces dried apricots, chopped
1 large apple, peeled, cored, and chopped
3 tablespoons apple juice plus 2 tablespoons water
1 vanilla bean (optional)
1 large pear, peeled, cored, and chopped

Put the apricots and apple into a heavy-bottomed saucepan together with the apple juice and water. Split the vanilla bean (if using), scrape the seeds into the pan, and throw in the split bean. Bring to a boil, then cover and simmer for 4 minutes. Add the chopped pear and continue to simmer for 2 minutes. Remove the vanilla bean. Puree in a blender.

Food fact: Dried apricots are one of nature's superfoods. The drying process concentrates the goodness of the original fruit. Dried apricots are an excellent source of iron—food for the brain. They are also rich in vitamins A and C, and have oodles of powerful potassium. Avoid dried apricots treated with sulfur dioxide, as these can trigger asthma or allergies in susceptible babies. Sulfur dioxide is used to keep the bright orange color, so it's best to choose darker brown dried apricots.

6–7 MONTHS

MAKES 4 PORTIONS

COOKING TIME: 6 MINUTES

SUITABLE FOR FREEZING

Serve this on its own or mix it with some baby rice cereal, yogurt, or mashed banana. Adding a vanilla bean gives the fruit a lovely flavor.

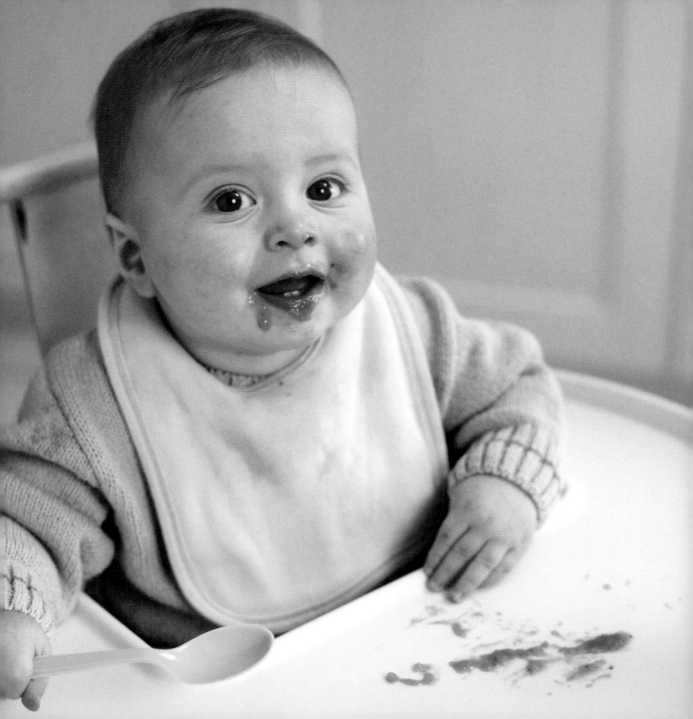

Second-stage weaning: 7 to 9 months

Once your baby can sit unsupported, he can use a high chair. Try to make eating a social event by getting him to sit at the table with you.

Foods with a thicker consistency and lumpier texture can be introduced to encourage your baby to learn to chew. If he is not hungry at mealtimes, cut down on the amount of milk he drinks so that he is hungrier for his solids and therefore not so fussy about the texture. Your baby should still be having a minimum of 18 to 20 ounces of milk a day.

Try to give 2 to 3 servings a day of starchy foods like potatoes, rice, pasta, or bread. Fruits and vegetables make good finger foods (see below) and should be included in at least two meals a day. Your baby should have one serving of cooked meat, fish, egg, or beans or lentils a day. It is important to include red meat in the diet, as it is an excellent source of iron. In addition, well-cooked eggs provide an excellent and cheap source of protein, as well as being very easy to prepare.

Once your baby can hold things in his hand, you can also give finger foods, such as:

- peeled apple, pear, or banana
- seedless grapes
- dried fruit—raisins or apricots
- steamed or raw vegetables—sticks of carrot or cucumber, broccoli florets
- cubes of cheese
- fingers of toast
- mini sandwiches
- rice cakes

7–9 MONTHS

MAKES 5 PORTIONS

COOKING TIME: 25 MINUTES

SUITABLE FOR FREEZING

Lentils can be difficult for young babies to digest and should be combined with plenty of fresh vegetables, as in this recipe. You can transform this tasty puree into a delicious soup for the family simply by adding more stock and some seasoning.

TOP TIP
A vegetarian baby's first tastes of food are the same as for other babies—baby rice, fruit and vegetable purees, etc. But from around seven months, when proteins are being introduced, the diet differs. Instead of meat, give dairy foods, eggs, and lentils. It's not as easy to absorb iron from nonanimal sources, so it's a good idea to give vitamin C–rich fruit or diluted juice to boost iron absorption.

Lovely lentils

½ cup finely chopped onion
2 medium carrots, peeled and chopped
2 tablespoons chopped celery
1 tablespoon vegetable oil
¼ cup split red lentils
1 medium sweet potato (8 ounces), peeled and chopped
1¾ cups Vegetable or Chicken Stock
    (see pages 124 and 125) or water

Sauté the onion, carrots, and celery in the vegetable oil for about 5 minutes or until softened. Add the lentils and sweet potato and pour in the stock or water . Bring to a boil, turn down the heat, and simmer, covered, for 20 minutes. Puree in a blender.

Food fact: Lentils are a good, cheap source of protein. They also provide iron, which is very important for brain development, particularly between the ages of six months and two years.

Potatoes blend well with most vegetables. Peel them just before cooking—don't soak them in water beforehand, as they will then lose their vitamin C.

Potato, leek, carrot, and peas

2 tablespoons unsalted butter
1 cup washed and sliced white part of a leek
2 small potatoes (6 ounces), peeled and cubed
1 medium carrot, peeled and sliced
1¼ cups Vegetable or Chicken Stock
   (see pages 124 and 125)
½ cup frozen peas

Melt the butter in a saucepan and sauté the leek for 3 to 4 minutes. Add the potatoes and carrot and pour in the stock. Bring to a boil, then reduce the heat, cover, and cook for 10 minutes. Add the frozen peas and continue to cook for about 6 minutes or until the vegetables are tender. For best results, puree in a food mill or blender rather than in a food processor.

Food fact: Potatoes contain vitamin C and are a good source of potassium.

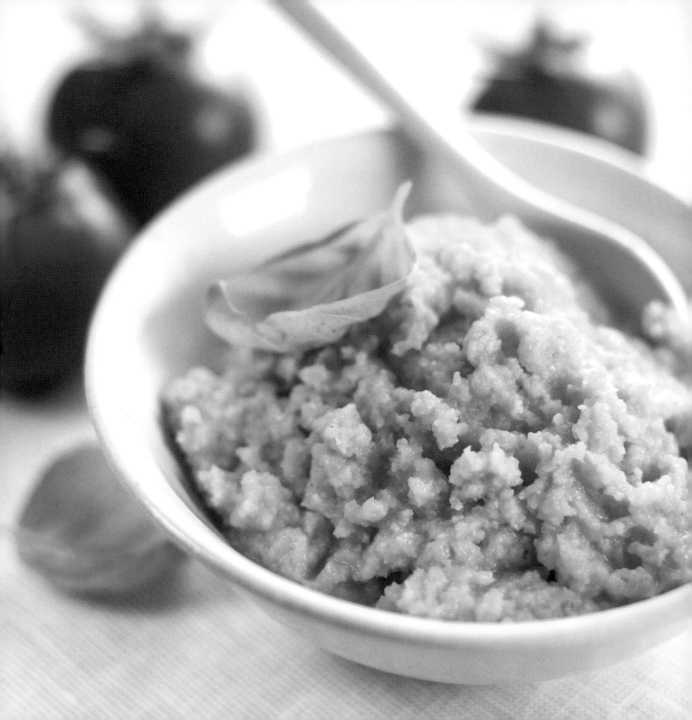

7–9 MONTHS

MAKES 4 PORTIONS

COOKING TIME: 18 MINUTES

SUITABLE FOR FREEZING

Tomato, cauliflower, and carrot with basil

2 medium carrots, peeled and sliced
1 cup chopped cauliflower florets
2 tablespoons unsalted butter
2 medium tomatoes (8 ounces), peeled, seeded,
*   and roughly chopped (see page 126)*
2 or 3 fresh basil leaves
½ cup grated Cheddar cheese

Put the carrots in a small saucepan, cover with boiling water, and simmer, covered, for 10 minutes. Add the cauliflower and cook, covered, for 7 to 8 minutes, adding extra water if necessary. Meanwhile, melt the butter in another pan, add the tomatoes, and sauté until mushy. Remove from the heat and stir in the basil and cheese until melted. Puree the carrots and cauliflower with the tomato sauce and about 3 tablespoons of the cooking liquid.

If you introduce your baby to new flavors at an early age, he will tend to grow up a less fussy eater. The sweet/tangy flavors of carrot and tomato in this recipe combine well with the mild-tasting cauliflower.

It's a good idea to introduce your child to the flavor of green vegetables early on. Since young babies can find certain vegetables too strong-tasting, you could try mixing these with something milder, such as combining broccoli with potato. You could also make this puree using sweet potato instead of white potato. For a tasty version mix ½ cup grated Cheddar cheese with the cooked vegetables and then puree.

Eat your greens

⅓ cup chopped onion
1 tablespoon unsalted butter
2 medium potatoes (8 ounces), peeled and cubed
1½ cups Vegetable Stock (see page 124) or water
½ cup chopped broccoli florets
¼ cup frozen peas
½ cup fresh spinach, washed and tough stems removed

Sauté the onion in the butter for about 5 minutes or until softened but not browned. Add the potatoes to the pan and pour in the stock or water. Cover, bring to a boil, and cook for 10 minutes. Add the broccoli florets and cook for 3 minutes, then add the peas and spinach and cook for 3 more minutes. Puree with as much of the cooking liquid as needed to make the desired consistency for your baby.

Mini minestrone

7–9 MONTHS

MAKES 3 PORTIONS

COOKING TIME: 28 MINUTES

SUITABLE FOR FREEZING

1 tablespoon vegetable oil
½ cup diced onion
1 clove garlic, crushed
½ cup diced carrot
¼ cup diced celery
¼ cup green beans, topped and tailed
   and cut into short lengths
½ cup diced potato
1 teaspoon tomato puree
1 cup Vegetable or Chicken Stock
   (see pages 124 and 125)
2 tablespoons small pasta stars
¼ cup frozen peas
1 tablespoon grated Parmesan cheese

The vegetables in minestrone soup add texture while being sufficiently soft for older babies to chew, as long as they are diced (as here). However, for younger babies you could blend this soup to the desired consistency.

Heat the oil in a saucepan and sauté the onion and garlic for 1 minute. Add the carrot and celery and continue to fry for 5 minutes. Add the beans, potato, and tomato puree and cook for 2 minutes. Pour in the stock, bring to a boil, and then simmer for 10 minutes. Add the pasta stars and cook for 5 minutes. Finally, add the peas and cook for 5 minutes more. Stir in the cheese. For younger babies, puree in a blender.

It's important to make sure that as well as fruits, vegetables, carbohydrates, and protein, babies have enough fat in their diet, as this is crucial for growth and development. Babies and young children need proportionately more fat in their diet than do adults. For this reason, dishes like vegetables in a cheese sauce or fruit with yogurt are ideal for your baby.

Vegetable puree with tomato and cheese

3 medium carrots, peeled and chopped
1 cup chopped cauliflower florets
⅓ cup sliced zucchini
1 tablespoon unsalted butter
*2 medium tomatoes (8 ounces), peeled, seeded,
    and chopped (see page 126)*
½ cup grated Cheddar cheese

Put the carrots into a steamer and cook for 10 minutes. If you have a multilayered steamer, place the cauliflower and zucchini in the basket above the carrots (otherwise, mix with the carrots) and continue to cook for 7 to 8 minutes. If you don't have a steamer, place the carrots in a saucepan, cover with water, and boil for 12 minutes. Add the cauliflower and zucchini and continue boiling for 7 to 8 minutes.

Meanwhile, melt the butter in a pan, add the chopped tomatoes, and sauté them for about 2 minutes or until slightly mushy. Remove from the heat and stir in the grated cheese until melted. Blend the carrots together with the cauliflower and zucchini, and mix together with the cheese and tomato sauce.

Vegetables with cheese sauce

7–9 MONTHS

MAKES 4 PORTIONS

COOKING TIME: 18 MINUTES

SUITABLE FOR FREEZING

1 medium carrot, peeled and sliced
1 cup chopped cauliflower florets
½ cup chopped broccoli florets
¼ cup frozen peas

Cheese sauce
1 tablespoon unsalted butter
1 tablespoon all-purpose flour
1 cup milk
⅓ cup grated Cheddar cheese

Put the carrot into a steamer set over a pan of boiling water, steam for 10 minutes, and set aside. Steam the cauliflower and broccoli for 4 minutes. Add the frozen peas and continue to cook for 3 minutes. Meanwhile, make the cheese sauce (see page 126).

Transfer the vegetables to a blender, pour in the sauce, and puree; or, for older babies, chop the vegetables and mix with the sauce. For young babies you can add a little more milk to thin the puree, if necessary. Spoon a little into your baby's bowl and serve lukewarm.

If your baby isn't too keen on eating his vegetables, try mixing them with a tasty cheese sauce.

TOP TIP
If you want to bring up your baby on a vegetarian diet, try to ensure that the diet is not too bulky—don't give too many high-fiber cereals and foods like lentils. Make sure that you provide plenty of high-calorie, nutrient-dense foods like cheese and eggs.

For the cheese sauce, you can experiment using different mild cheeses, like Edam or Emmental. You could also mix in other vegetables, like carrots or spinach.

Cauliflower and broccoli in cheese sauce

1¼ cups chopped cauliflower florets
½ cup chopped broccoli florets

Cheese sauce
1 tablespoon unsalted butter
1 tablespoon all-purpose flour
1 cup milk
Pinch of freshly grated nutmeg
3 tablespoons grated Cheddar cheese
2 tablespoons grated Gruyère cheese

Steam the cauliflower and broccoli for about 7 minutes or until tender (or boil in a saucepan of water for 7 minutes or until tender). Meanwhile, prepare the cheese sauce as instructed on page 126, adding the nutmeg with the milk and adding both cheeses to the sauce. Puree in a blender for babies under nine months. For older babies able to chew, chop the cauliflower and broccoli into small pieces and mix with the cheese sauce.

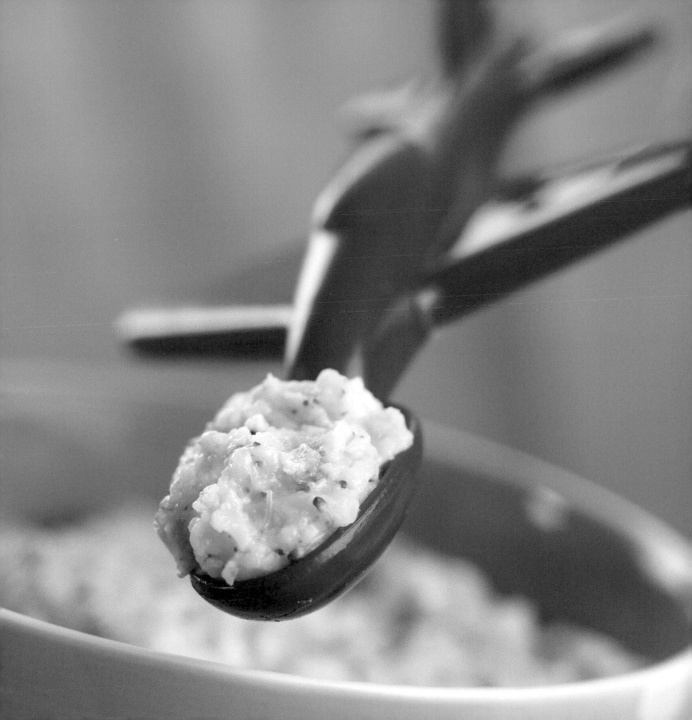

Butternut squash is very popular with young babies because of its smooth texture and naturally sweet taste.

Pasta with butternut squash, tomato, and cheese

1 small butternut squash (8 ounces), chopped
1½ tablespoons tiny pasta stars
1 tablespoon unsalted butter
2 medium tomatoes (8 ounces), peeled, seeded, and chopped (see page 126)
¼ cup grated Cheddar cheese
2 tablespoons milk

Steam or boil the butternut squash for 10 minutes or until tender. Meanwhile, cook the pasta stars according to the instructions on the package, but without adding salt to the water. Melt the butter in a small saucepan and sauté the tomatoes until mushy, then stir in the cheese until melted. Blend the cooked butternut squash and tomato and cheese mixture together with the milk using a handheld electric blender, and stir in the pasta stars.

7–9 MONTHS

MAKES 5 PORTIONS

COOKING TIME: 20 MINUTES

SUITABLE FOR FREEZING

This is one of my family's favorite fish recipes. Do not be put off by the odd-sounding combination, as it gives a marvelously rich taste.

Fillet of fish in an orange sauce

8 ounces haddock or flounder fillets, skinned
½ cup orange juice
⅓ cup grated Cheddar cheese
1 tablespoon finely chopped fresh parsley
2 tablespoons crushed cornflakes
1 tablespoon unsalted butter

Put the fish in a greased dish, cover with the orange juice, cheese, parsley, and cornflakes, and dot with the butter. Cover with foil and bake at 350°F for about 20 minutes. Alternatively, cover with microwave-safe plastic wrap and cook in a microwave on high for 4 minutes. Flake the fish carefully, removing any bones, and mash everything together with the liquid in which the fish was cooked.

Flounder is one of the best fish to start with, as it has a suitably soft texture for young babies.

Fillet of flounder with carrot, cheese, and tomato

4 medium carrots, peeled and sliced
8 ounces flounder fillets, skinned
2 tablespoons milk
3 tablespoons unsalted butter
2 medium tomatoes (8 ounces), peeled, seeded, and chopped
(see page 126)
⅓ cup grated Cheddar cheese

Put the carrots in a steamer set over a pan of boiling water and cook for 15 minutes. Meanwhile, place the fish in a microwave dish, add the milk, dot with 1 tablespoon of the butter, and cover, leaving an air vent. Microwave on high for 2 to 3 minutes. Alternatively, put the fish in a pan, cover with a little milk, add 1 tablespoon of the butter, and simmer for 3 to 4 minutes or until cooked.

Melt the remaining 2 tablespoons butter in a saucepan, add the tomatoes, and sauté until mushy. Stir in the cheese until melted. Blend the carrots with the tomato mixture. Remove the fish from its cooking liquor and flake, making sure there are no bones. Mix the fish with the carrots and tomatoes. For younger babies you can blend the fish together with the carrots and tomato for a smoother texture.

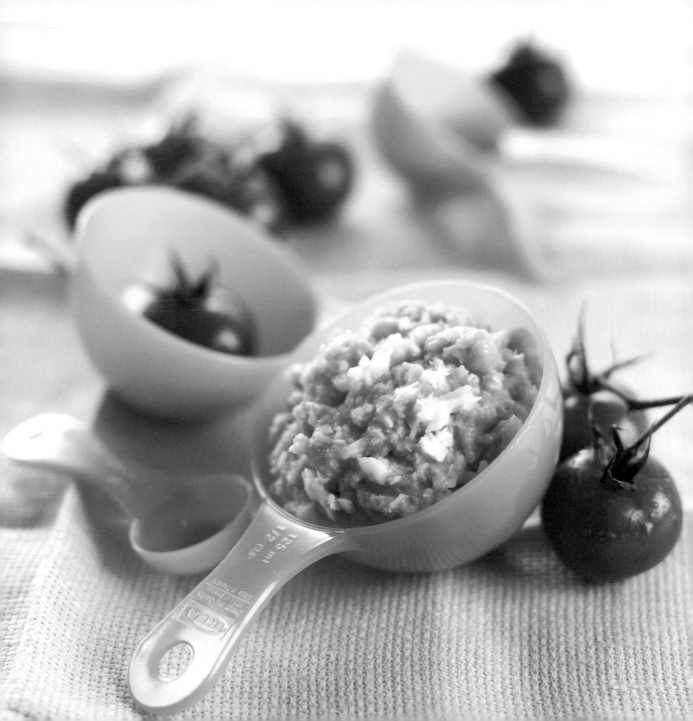

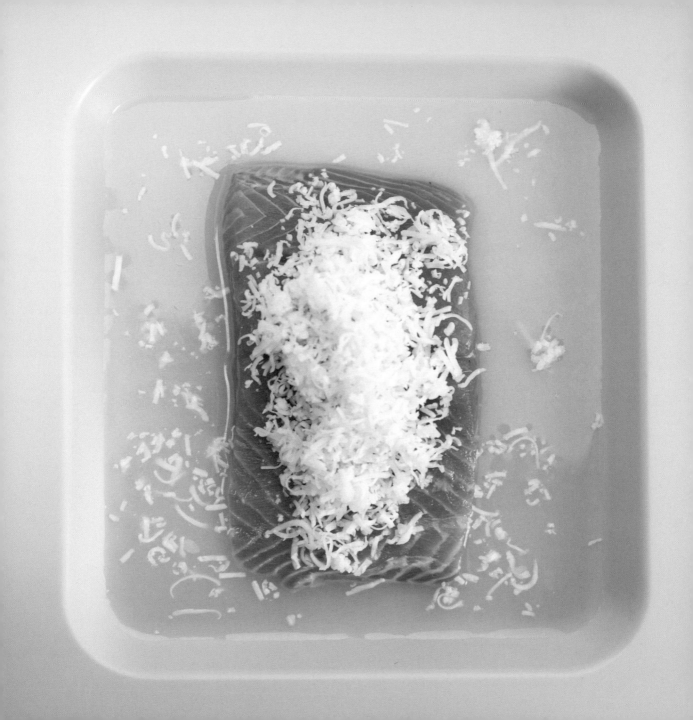

Salmon surprise

2 medium carrots, peeled and sliced
4½ ounces salmon fillet, skinned
¼ cup orange juice
⅓ cup grated Cheddar cheese
1 tablespoon unsalted butter
2 tablespoons milk

Put the carrots into a saucepan, cover with water, bring to a boil, and cook over medium heat for about 20 minutes or until tender. Alternatively, place the vegetables in a steamer and cook for 20 minutes.

Meanwhile, place the salmon in a suitable dish, pour in the orange juice, and scatter the cheese on top. Cover, leaving an air vent, and microwave on high for about 2 minutes or until the fish flakes easily with a fork. Alternatively, cover with foil and cook in the oven, preheated to 350°F, for about 20 minutes.

Flake the fish with a fork, carefully removing any bones. Drain the carrots, mix with the butter and milk, and puree in a blender together with the flaked fish and its sauce. For older babies, mash the carrots together with the butter and the milk and then mix the flaked fish with the mashed carrots.

Food fact: Oily fish like salmon provides a good source of essential fatty acids that are important for development of the brain and eyes.

7–9 MONTHS

MAKES 3 PORTIONS

COOKING TIME: 20 MINUTES

SUITABLE FOR FREEZING

Like the previous recipe, this also uses the delicious, if slightly unusual, combination of fish and orange.

Babies love the sweet taste of corn. The trouble is, when it is made into a puree the kernels tend to be a bit lumpy and difficult to digest, so for young babies I prefer to put it through a food mill. For older babies, I puree the potato mixture and then stir in the corn whole.

Cherub's chowder

1 onion, chopped
1 tablespoon vegetable oil
2 medium potatoes (8 ounces), peeled and diced
¾ cup Vegetable or Chicken Stock
    (see pages 124 and 125)
⅓ cup canned or frozen corn
¼ cup milk
½ cup diced cooked chicken

Sauté the chopped onion in the oil until soft. Add the potatoes to the pan and pour in the stock. Bring to a boil, then cover and simmer for about 12 minutes. Add the corn and the milk and simmer for 2 to 3 more minutes. Puree the soup in a food mill, together with the chicken, and heat through. Alternatively, for older babies, puree the onion and potato mixture in a food mill, then stir in the corn whole and the chicken. Add a little extra milk and stock to make this into soup.

Chicken liver with vegetables and apple

7–9 MONTHS

MAKES 5 PORTIONS

COOKING TIME: 23 MINUTES

SUITABLE FOR FREEZING

4 ounces chicken livers
⅓ cup chopped onion
1 tablespoon vegetable oil
1 medium carrot, peeled and sliced
1 large potato, peeled and cubed
½ small apple, peeled, cored, and chopped
1 cup Chicken Stock (see page 125)

Clean the livers, removing any fat or gristle, and slice them. Sauté the onion in the vegetable oil until softened. Add the sliced liver and sauté for about 1 minute or until it has changed color. Add the carrot, potato, and apple, pour in the stock, and simmer for 20 minutes. Puree in a food processor.

Food fact: Chicken liver provides a good source of vitamins and iron. Babies are born with a store of iron that lasts for about six months, so after this time it is important to ensure they get all the iron that they need from their diet.

TOP TIP
When teething, your baby may lose his appetite. Rubbing a teething gel onto his gums may help ease the pain. It can also be soothing for your baby to chew on something cool, like a chilled cucumber stick.

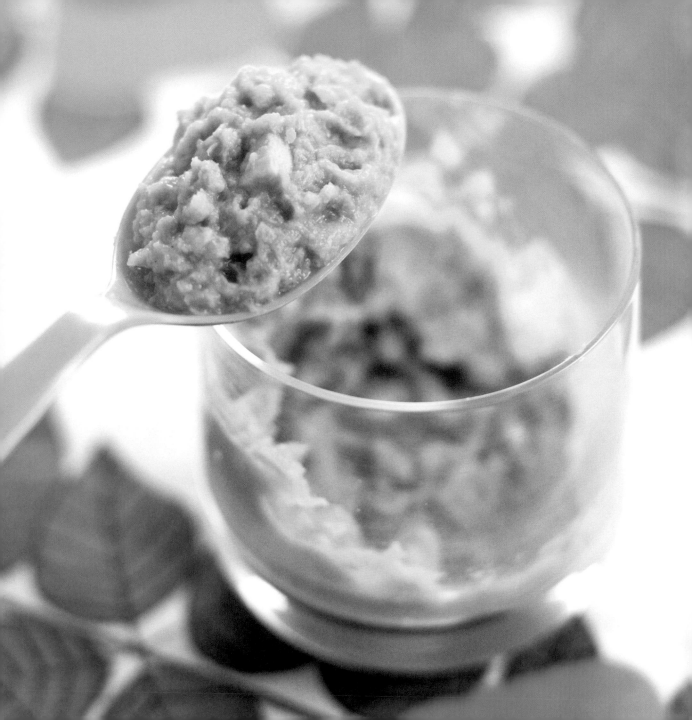

🍼 7–9 MONTHS

🥣 MAKES 2 PORTIONS

🕐 COOKING TIME: 28–30 MINUTES

❄️ SUITABLE FOR FREEZING

Chicken with leek, carrot, and peas

Since the dark meat of a chicken is even more nutritious than the breast, and tends to be moister, it's a good idea sometimes to use the thighs instead.

1½ teaspoons vegetable oil
⅓ cup washed and chopped white part of a leek
1 large chicken thigh (about 6 ounces) on the bone, skinned and trimmed of fat
2 medium carrots, peeled and chopped
1 cup Chicken Stock (see page 125)
¼ cup frozen peas

Heat the oil in a saucepan and sauté the leek for 2 minutes. Add the chicken and sauté for about 2 minutes. Add the carrots and pour in the stock, then bring to a boil, cover, and simmer for 20 minutes. Add the peas and cook uncovered for 4 to 5 minutes. Remove the chicken with a slotted spoon and take the flesh off the bone. Blend together the vegetables and chicken with as much of the cooking liquid as necessary to make a smooth puree.

Beef needs long, slow cooking to make it really tender.

My first beef casserole

1½ tablespoons vegetable oil
1 onion, finely chopped
1 clove garlic, crushed
1½ tablespoons all-purpose flour
1 teaspoon paprika
11 ounces lean stewing beef
1¾ cups Chicken Stock (see page 125) or water
2 medium carrots, peeled and chopped
3 medium potatoes (12 ounces), peeled and chopped
½ stalk celery, trimmed and chopped
Sprig of parsley
Sprig of thyme (optional)
¾ cup wiped and sliced button mushrooms

Preheat the oven to 300°F. Heat the oil in a casserole dish and sauté the onion and garlic for 3 minutes. Mix the flour and paprika together in a small bowl and toss the meat in this to coat it. Add the floured meat to the casserole and sauté until browned all over.

Pour in the stock or water and stir for 1 minute. Add the vegetables and herbs, then cover and cook in the preheated oven for 2 hours. Add the mushrooms and continue to cook for 30 minutes. Puree in a blender.

Food fact: Red meat provides the richest source of iron, which is essential for your baby's physical and mental development.

Braised beef with carrot, parsnip, and sweet potato

7–9 MONTHS

MAKES 5 PORTIONS

COOKING TIME:
1 HOUR 50 MINUTES

SUITABLE FOR FREEZING

1 tablespoon olive oil
½ cup chopped red onion
1 clove garlic, crushed
5 ounces lean beef, cut into pieces
2 tablespoons all-purpose flour
2 medium carrots, peeled and sliced
1 small parsnip (3 ounces), peeled and sliced
1 medium sweet potato (8 ounces), peeled and chopped
1 bay leaf
1 tablespoon chopped fresh parsley
1¾ cups Chicken Stock (see page 125)

This recipe makes a good introduction to red meat. Sometimes babies don't like to eat it because they find it too difficult to chew. In this recipe, I have mixed the meat together with root vegetables to give the meat a smooth texture and a flavor that will appeal to babies.

Heat the oil in a heavy-bottomed saucepan or small casserole dish. Sauté the onion and garlic for 3 to 4 minutes or until softened. Toss the pieces of beef in the flour and sauté until browned all over. Add the carrots, parsnip, sweet potato, bay leaf, and parsley to the pan and pour in the stock. Bring to a boil and then simmer, covered, for about 1¾ hours or until the meat is tender. Blend, adding as much of the cooking liquid as necessary.

Lamb tends to be quite
popular with young babies,
and combining lamb with
sweet potato gives it a nice
soft texture.

Sweet potato and lamb casserole

One 3½-ounce lamb chop, trimmed of fat and diced
2 scallions, thinly sliced
1 large sweet potato (10 to 12 ounces),
    peeled and chopped
1 medium tomato (4 ounces), peeled, seeded,
    and chopped (see page 126)
Pinch of dried rosemary or mixed herbs
½ cup Chicken Stock (see page 125)

Preheat the oven to 350°F. Put all the ingredients
into a small casserole dish, cover, and bake for
10 to 15 minutes or until bubbling. Reduce the heat
to 300°F and continue to cook for about 45 minutes
or until the lamb is tender. Blend to a puree or chop
into small pieces for older babies.

Food fact: Lamb provides a good source of B vitamins,
zinc, and iron.

Baby muesli

2 tablespoons rolled oats
1 tablespoon finely chopped dried apricots
1½ teaspoons raisins
1 tablespoon ground almonds
¼ cup apple, orange, or pineapple juice
½ small apple, peeled, cored, and grated

Mix together the oats, apricots, raisins, and ground almonds in the plastic bowl of a handheld electric blender. Pour in the juice and leave to soak for 5 minutes. When softened, blend to make a finer texture, then stir in the grated apple.

FROM 8 MONTHS

MAKES 1 PORTION

COOKING TIME: NONE

UNSUITABLE FOR FREEZING

This tasty and nutritious breakfast will make a good start to the day for your baby. You can also add other fruits, like chopped peach or banana. Omit the ground almonds if there is any history of allergy in the family.

Oatmeal with banana

½ cup milk
3 tablespoons instant oatmeal
1 small banana
1 teaspoon maple syrup or a sprinkling of brown sugar

Bring the milk to a boil in a small saucepan. Stir in the instant oatmeal and cook over low heat until thickened. Mash the banana and stir into the cereal, together with the maple syrup or sugar.

7–9 MONTHS

MAKES 1 PORTION

COOKING TIME: 5 MINUTES

UNSUITABLE FOR FREEZING

You don't need to give only special baby cereals to your child; the cereal should contain less than 1g salt per serving. You could crush a shredded wheat biscuit and mix it with milk and mashed banana.

7–9 MONTHS

MAKES 4 PORTIONS

COOKING TIME: 3 MINUTES

SUITABLE FOR FREEZING

This was my children's favorite breakfast when they were babies. Not only does it taste great, it is also packed full of nutritious ingredients.

TOP TIP
Your baby may start grabbing the spoon you use to feed her, so it's a good idea to give her a second, identical spoon to hold while you feed her. Once she can get the spoon into her mouth, try giving her food that will stick to the spoon, like oatmeal.

My favorite oatmeal

½ cup milk
¼ cup rolled oats
6 dried apricots, chopped
1 large pear, peeled, cored, and chopped

Put the milk, oatmeal, and chopped apricots into a small saucepan, bring to a boil, and then simmer, stirring occasionally, for 3 minutes. Puree with the chopped pear using a handheld electric blender.

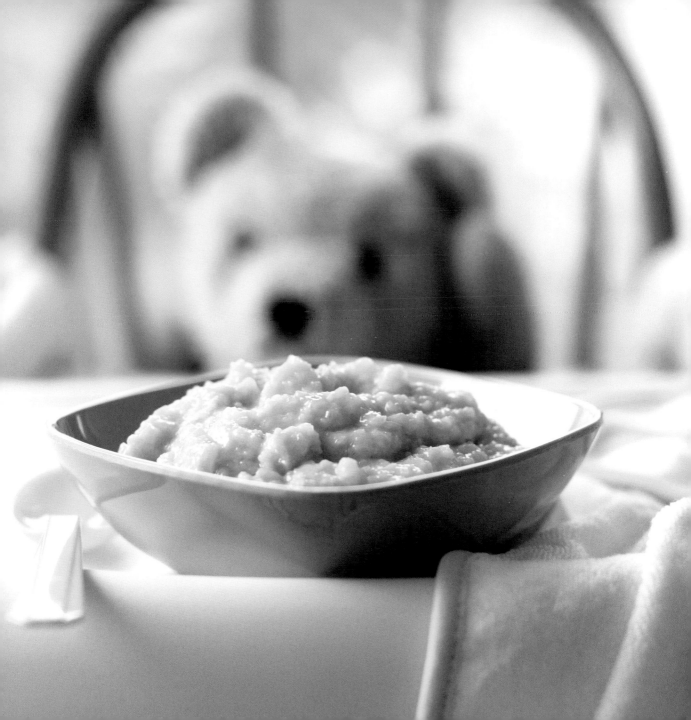

You could also make this recipe using soft, ready-to-eat dried figs instead of prunes.

Apple, pear, and prune with oats

2 tablespoons rolled oats
¼ cup unsweetened apple juice
2 tablespoons water
1 small apple, peeled, cored, and chopped
2 pitted prunes, chopped
1 small pear, peeled, cored, and chopped

Put the oats, apple juice, and water in a saucepan, bring to a boil, and simmer for 2 minutes. Add the apple, prunes, and pear, cover, and simmer for 3 minutes, stirring occasionally. Puree to the desired consistency.

Food fact: Prunes are a good source of instant energy, fiber, and iron. They help with constipation, as they are a natural laxative.

Apple and mango

2 medium apples, peeled, cored, and chopped
2 tablespoons apple juice or water
½ cup chopped mango

Put the chopped apples into a heavy-bottomed saucepan together with the apple juice or water and cook over low heat for about 6 minutes. Puree in a blender together with the mango.

Food fact: Mangoes are a rich source of vitamin A, which is essential for healthy skin, eyesight, and fighting infection. They are also rich in vitamin C, which boosts immunity and helps our bodies to absorb iron. If your baby is having tummy troubles, mangoes may help, as they are highly alkaline and can balance out any acidity in your baby's stomach. Mangoes also contain calcium and magnesium, which are good for building strong bones and teeth.

7–9 MONTHS

MAKES 3 PORTIONS

COOKING TIME: 6 MINUTES

SUITABLE FOR FREEZING

This puree takes just minutes to prepare and is delicious when you have a ripe mango; when a mango is ripe, the skin will give slightly when you push it, and the mango should also smell fragrant.

In the summer, when cherries are deliciously sweet, it's nice to be able to give them to your baby.

Banana and cherry

6 sweet cherries, halved and pitted
1 tablespoon water
1 banana
1 tablespoon baby rice cereal

Put the cherries into a small pan together with the water and simmer for 2 minutes. Mash the banana, add to the cooked cherries, and simmer for just under a minute. Puree using a handheld electric blender and stir in the baby rice.

Food fact: Cherries stimulate the immune system and help to prevent infection. They are also good for a child suffering from constipation.

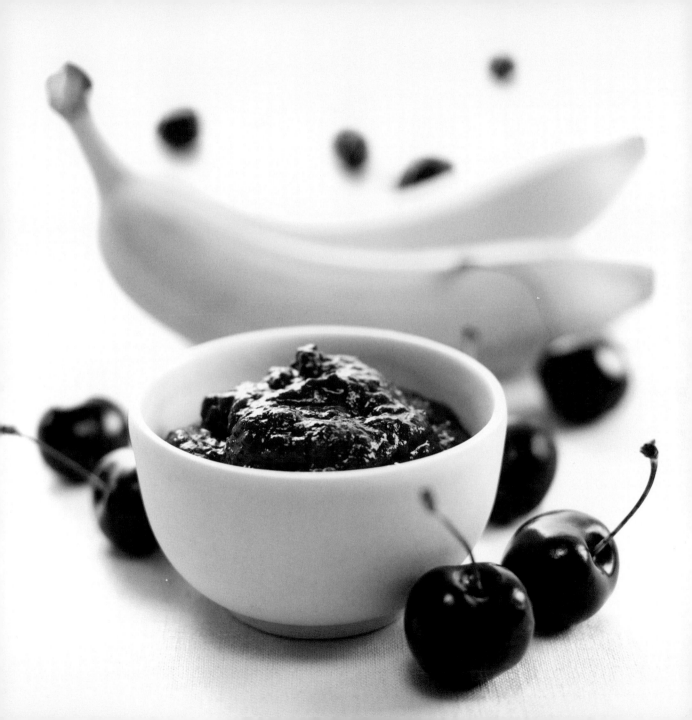

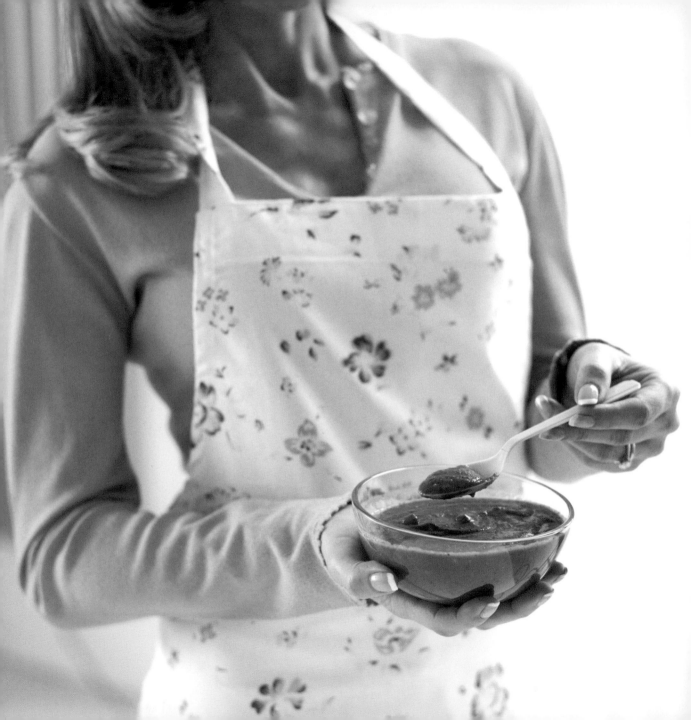

Blueberry, banana, and apple

1 cup blueberries
1 small banana, sliced
1 small apple, peeled, cored, and chopped

Put all the fruit into a heavy-bottomed pan and cook, covered, over low heat for 5 minutes. Uncover and simmer for 5 minutes more or until most of the juices have evaporated.

7–9 MONTHS

MAKES 3 PORTIONS

COOKING TIME: 10 MINUTES

UNSUITABLE FOR FREEZING

Strawberry, peach, and pear crumble

⅓ cup hulled and quartered strawberries
1 large, juicy peach, peeled, pitted, and
    cut into pieces (see page 126)
1 large pear, peeled, cored, and cut into pieces
1 zwieback

Put the fruit into a small, heavy-bottomed saucepan, cover, and simmer for about 3 minutes. Crush the zwieback (place in a plastic bag and crush with a rolling pin), then blend it together with the fruit.

7–9 MONTHS

MAKES 2 PORTIONS

COOKING TIME: 3 MINUTES

SUITABLE FOR FREEZING

Some fruit purees are very runny, but you can thicken them by stirring in some baby rice, mashed banana, or crumbled zwieback, as here. You could also make this with 2 peaches instead of the pear.

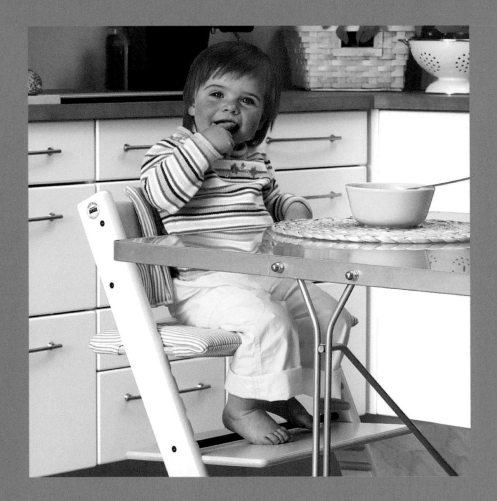

Growing independence: 9 to 12 months

The final quarter of a baby's first year is a period of rapid change. She will progress from sitting to crawling and maybe even walking. This is a time of growing independence, and you may find that your baby will increasingly insist on feeding herself.

Offer finger foods as part of her meals to give chewing practice and to encourage her to feed herself if she is not doing so already. Give steamed or raw vegetable sticks or fresh fruit with a favorite fruit puree as a dip. (See page 63 for other suggestions.)

Her diet can now include virtually all the same foods eaten by the rest of the family, except added salt, lightly cooked eggs, unpasteurized cheeses, low-fat or high-fiber products, whole nuts, and honey.

If your baby is on the move, you may need to increase the amount of food you give to her. Make sure her diet includes full-fat dairy products, in addition to fruit and vegetables, and nutrient-dense foods like Tuna Pasta with Creamy Tomato Sauce or Risotto with Butternut Squash (pages 109 and 100). Babies only have small stomachs and so need to be fed at regular intervals.

Try to dispense with bottles by the time your baby is a year old, except for perhaps one at bedtime. Encourage your baby to drink from a cup or beaker—it is better for her teeth.

Eggs are quick to prepare but must be cooked through; raw or lightly cooked eggs should not be given to babies or young children because of the risk of salmonella. For babies under one year, the white and yolk should be cooked until solid. You could add some chopped tomato to the scrambled egg if you like.

Scrambled egg with cheese

2 eggs
1 tablespoon milk
2 tablespoons grated Cheddar cheese
1 tablespoon unsalted butter

Whisk together the eggs, milk, and cheese. Melt the butter in a small pan, add the egg mixture, and then cook over low heat for 2 to 3 minutes, stirring, until the mixture sets.

Food fact: Eggs provide protein, vitamins, and minerals, while egg yolk offers a good source of iron for your baby.

Carrot, cheese, and tomato risotto

😊 9–12 MONTHS

🥣 MAKES 4 PORTIONS

🕐 COOKING TIME: 20–25 MINUTES

❄ SUITABLE FOR FREEZING

¼ cup chopped onion
1 tablespoon unsalted butter
½ cup long-grain rice
2 medium carrots, peeled and sliced
1¼ cups boiling water
2 medium tomatoes (8 ounces), peeled, seeded, and
    chopped (see page 126)
½ cup grated Cheddar cheese

Sauté the onion in half the butter until softened. Stir in the rice until well coated, then add the carrots. Pour in the boiling water, bring back to a boil, then cover the pan and simmer for 15 to 20 minutes or until the rice is cooked and the carrots are tender. If necessary, add extra water.

Meanwhile, melt the remaining butter in a small pan, add the tomatoes, and sauté for 2 to 3 minutes or until mushy. Stir in the cheese until melted. The water from the rice should have been absorbed, but if not, drain off any excess. Stir the tomato and cheese mixture into the cooked rice.

This dish is both nutritious and very easy to prepare. Cooked rice is soft, so it is a good way of introducing texture to your baby's food. Babies and toddlers tend to like rice and carrots, and here I have flavored them with sautéed tomatoes and melted cheese for a very tasty meal.

TOP TIP
Surveys have shown that 1 in every 5 babies aged 10 to 12 months has a daily intake of iron below the recommended level.

Serving cooked rice with vegetables is an ideal way to introduce texture to your baby's food. Butternut squash is now more readily available in supermarkets, although you could substitute pumpkin instead.

TOP TIP
The more you allow your baby to experiment using a spoon, the quicker she will learn to feed herself.

Risotto with butternut squash

½ cup chopped onion
1 tablespoon unsalted butter
½ cup basmati rice
2 cups boiling water
½ medium butternut squash (6 ounces),
    peeled and chopped
2 medium tomatoes (8 ounces), peeled, seeded, and
    chopped (see page 126)
½ cup grated Cheddar cheese

Sauté the onion in half the butter until softened. Stir in the rice until well coated. Pour in the boiling water, cover the pan, and cook for 8 minutes over high heat. Stir in the butternut squash, reduce the heat, and cook, covered, for about 12 minutes or until the water has been absorbed.

Meanwhile, melt the remaining butter in a small saucepan, add the tomatoes, and sauté for 2 to 3 minutes. Stir in the cheese until melted, then stir the tomato and cheese mixture into the cooked rice.

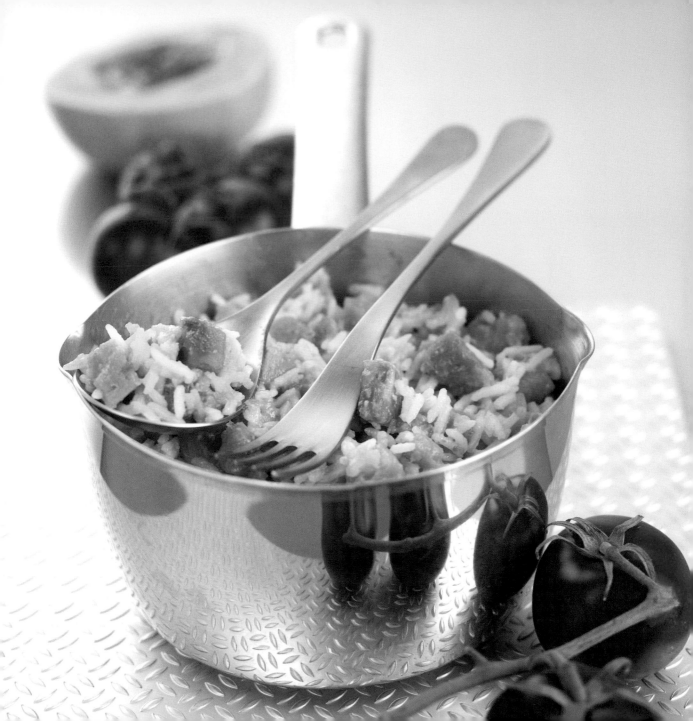

Pasta is a great energy food. Orzo are tiny pasta shapes that look like rice, but if you can't find them, you could use any other small pasta shapes instead. You can vary the vegetables, if you like, using peas and corn instead of zucchini and broccoli, and adding diced tomatoes with the cheese.

Pasta risotto

½ cup orzo or other small pasta shapes
1 small carrot, peeled and diced
1 small zucchini, diced
½ cup chopped broccoli florets
1 tablespoon unsalted butter
¼ cup grated Cheddar cheese

Put the pasta in a saucepan together with the carrot, cover generously with boiling water, and cook for 5 minutes. Add the zucchini and broccoli and continue to cook for about 7 minutes. Melt the butter in a saucepan, stir in the drained pasta and vegetables, and toss with the butter and Cheddar until the cheese has melted.

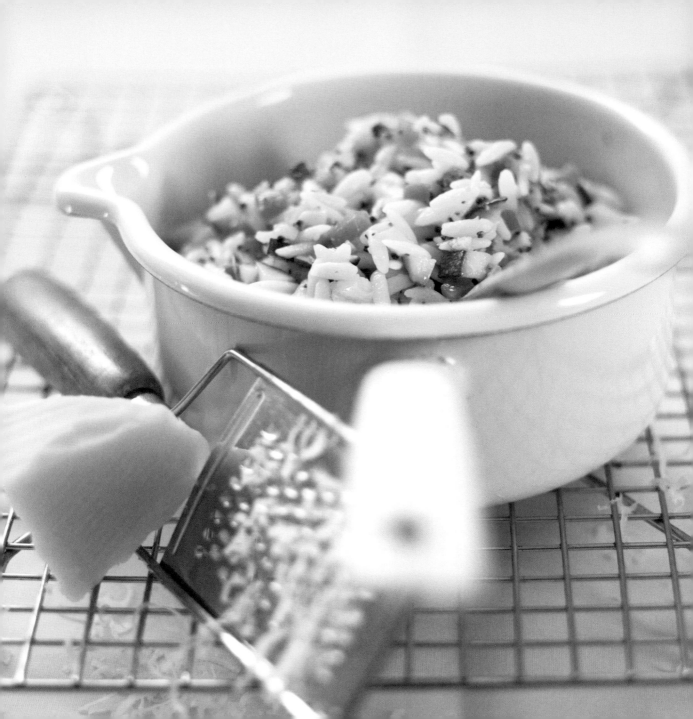

Adding tiny pasta shapes to purees introduces texture in a gradual way. This tasty sauce is also very nutritious.

Pasta stars with tasty vegetable sauce

1 tablespoon olive oil
½ cup chopped onion
1 clove garlic, crushed
2 medium carrots, peeled and chopped
⅓ cup chopped red bell pepper
Half a 15-ounce can diced tomatoes
1 cup water
3 tablespoons tiny pasta stars
2 tablespoons frozen peas
¼ cup grated Cheddar cheese

Heat the oil in a saucepan and sauté the onion and garlic for 1 minute. Add the carrots and bell pepper and continue to cook for 5 minutes. Add the tomatoes and water. Bring to a boil, then cover and simmer for 15 minutes.

Meanwhile, cook the pasta stars according to the instructions on the package, but without adding salt to the water. Add the peas to the tomatoes and vegetables and continue to cook for 5 minutes. Remove from the heat and stir in the grated cheese until melted. Blend the mixture to a puree. Drain the pasta and stir into the sauce.

Food fact: Tomatoes are rich in lycopene, a powerful antioxidant that helps protect against heart disease and cancer.

9–12 MONTHS

MAKES 4 PORTIONS

COOKING TIME: 20 MINUTES

SUITABLE FOR FREEZING

Mashed potato and carrot with broccoli and cheese

3 medium potatoes (12 ounces), peeled and chopped
2 medium carrots, peeled and sliced
½ cup chopped broccoli florets
2 tablespoons milk
1 tablespoon unsalted butter
¼ cup grated Cheddar cheese

Put the potatoes and carrots into a saucepan, cover with boiling water, and cook for about 20 minutes or until tender. Meanwhile, steam the broccoli for 7 to 8 minutes until tender. Alternatively, add to the potatoes and carrots after about 12 minutes and continue cooking for 7 to 8 minutes. Drain the potatoes and carrots and mash together with the broccoli, milk, butter, and cheese.

Mashing rather than pureeing your baby's food is a good way to gradually introduce more texture. The relatively strong flavor of the broccoli is toned down by the creamy mashed potatoes and cheese.

TOP TIP
A bowl that sticks to the tray of the high chair with suction is a good idea, as it makes it easier for your baby to get food onto his spoon without the bowl moving around on the tray.

This is a great way to get children to eat vegetables because they are blended into the sauce to make them invisible, and what they can't see, they can't pick out. For a creamier version, you can stir in a little mascarpone (an Italian cream cheese).

Pasta with hidden vegetables

2 tablespoons light olive oil
1 small onion, chopped
1 clove garlic, crushed
2 small carrots, peeled and chopped
1 medium zucchini, trimmed and chopped
¾ cup wiped and chopped button mushrooms
3 plum tomatoes, peeled, seeded, and chopped
   (see page 126)
1 tablespoon unsalted butter
One 15-ounce can diced tomatoes
½ cup Vegetable Stock (see page 124)
¼ teaspoon brown sugar
1 tablespoon torn fresh basil leaves
Freshly ground black pepper
6 ounces pasta shapes
3 to 4 tablespoons mascarpone cheese (optional)

Heat the oil in a saucepan, add the onion and garlic, and sauté for about 3 minutes. Add the carrots and sauté for 4 to 5 minutes. Add the zucchini and sauté for 2 minutes, followed by the mushrooms, sautéing for 2 minutes.

Add the fresh tomatoes and the butter and sauté for 2 minutes. Pour in the can of tomatoes and half the juice. Finally, add the stock, sugar, and basil, and season with pepper to taste. Cover and cook over medium heat for 10 minutes, then blend to a puree.

Meanwhile, cook the pasta according to the package instructions until tender, but without adding any salt. Toss the cooked pasta with the sauce and mascarpone (if using).

Spinach is a good source of beta-carotene and vitamin C, so try not to overcook it or you will destroy a lot of its vitamin content.

TOP TIP
If your baby is constipated, give foods that are naturally rich in fiber, like prunes, cooked pears, mashed papaya, lentils, and whole-grain cereals. Stop giving rice cereal or banana, and increase fluids wherever possible, in the form of breast milk, water, or diluted juice.

Fillet of cod with spinach in a cheese sauce

7 ounces cod fillet, skinned
1 tablespoon unsalted butter
½ lemon
1 cup fresh spinach, washed and tough stems removed

Cheese sauce
1 tablespoon unsalted butter
1 tablespoon all-purpose flour
¾ cup milk
Pinch of freshly grated nutmeg
¼ cup grated Cheddar cheese

Put the fish in a suitable dish, dot with the butter, and add a squeeze of lemon juice. Cover, leaving an air vent, and microwave on high for 3 to 4 minutes or until the fish flakes easily with a fork. Alternatively, you can poach the fish in the milk (for the cheese sauce) with a bay leaf, a parsley sprig, and a few peppercorns for 3 to 4 minutes, then strain the milk and use to make the cheese sauce.

Cook the spinach in a saucepan with just a little water clinging to the leaves for about 2 minutes or until wilted, and squeeze out any excess liquid. To make the cheese sauce, follow the instructions on page 126, adding the nutmeg with the milk. Flake the cooked fish, chop the spinach, and mix with the cheese sauce.

Tuna pasta with creamy tomato sauce

¼ cup small pasta shapes
¼ cup finely chopped onion
1 clove garlic, crushed
1 tablespoon vegetable oil
½ cup canned crushed tomatoes
One 6-ounce can tuna in oil, drained and flaked

Cheese sauce
1 tablespoon unsalted butter
1 tablespoon all-purpose flour
½ cup milk
¼ cup grated Cheddar cheese

Cook the pasta according to the package instructions, but without adding salt to the water. To make the cheese sauce, follow the instructions on page 126. Meanwhile, sauté the onion and garlic in the oil until softened, stir in the tomatoes and flaked tuna, and cook for about 4 minutes. Mix the cheese sauce with the tuna and tomato and stir in the cooked pasta.

Food fact: Tuna provides an excellent source of protein and vitamins, especially D and B_{12}. However, unlike fresh tuna, canned tuna does not contain omega-3 essential fatty acids.

9–12 MONTHS

MAKES 3 PORTIONS

COOKING TIME: 12 MINUTES

SUITABLE FOR FREEZING

Canned tuna is so nutritious and such a great cupboard standby that it's good to encourage a liking for it at an early age.

Mixing soft cooked rice or small pasta shapes into your baby's puree is a good way to introduce texture.

Chicken with tomato and rice

1 tablespoon olive oil
½ cup chopped onion
1 small clove garlic, crushed
3 ounces boneless, skinless chicken breast,
*   cut into chunks*
2 medium carrots, peeled and chopped
2 medium potatoes (8 ounces), peeled and chopped
Half a 15-ounce can diced tomatoes
Sprig of thyme (optional)
½ cup Chicken Stock (see page 125) or water
¼ cup apple juice
¼ cup cooked rice

Heat the oil in a heavy-bottomed saucepan and sauté the onion and garlic for about 4 minutes or until softened but not browned. Add the chicken and sauté for about 2 minutes or until browned. Add the carrots, potatoes, tomatoes, and thyme (if using) and pour in the stock or water and the apple juice. Bring to a boil, then cover and simmer for 20 minutes.

Remove the thyme. Blitz the chicken and vegetables to the desired consistency in a blender, then mix in the cooked rice.

Tasty chicken Bolognese

9–12 MONTHS

MAKES 2 PORTIONS

COOKING TIME: 24 MINUTES

SUITABLE FOR FREEZING

This delicious sauce can be mixed with any type of pasta. As your baby gets older, you will probably find that you don't need to puree the sauce.

1 tablespoon olive oil
1 small onion, chopped
1 clove garlic, crushed
2 small carrots, peeled and grated
5 ounces ground chicken or turkey
½ teaspoon fresh thyme leaves or
    a pinch of dried thyme
½ cup canned crushed tomatoes
½ cup Chicken Stock (see page 125)
1 ounce spaghetti

Heat the oil in a saucepan, add the onion and garlic, and sauté for 3 minutes, stirring occasionally. Add the carrots and continue to cook for 3 minutes. Add the chicken and cook, stirring occasionally, for about 3 minutes. Add the thyme, tomatoes, and stock, bring to a boil, and then simmer, covered, for 15 minutes.

Meanwhile, cook the spaghetti according to the instructions on the package, without adding any salt. Drain and chop into small pieces. Using a handheld electric blender, whiz the Bolognese sauce for a few seconds to make a smoother texture and then stir in the chopped spaghetti.

Chicken is a good source of lean protein as well as having a suitably soft texture for your baby. The darker meat of chicken legs contains twice as much iron and zinc as the lighter meat.

TOP TIP
Once babies are eating a varied diet, you may find that some foods, such as raisins, may appear in your baby's stools in their original state. Don't worry; this is quite normal.

Chicken with corn and rice

2 chicken legs, skinned (about 9 ounces)
1 bay leaf
Sprig of parsley
3 black peppercorns
1¾ cups Chicken Stock (see page 125)
1 tablespoon unsalted butter
1 tablespoon all-purpose flour
¼ cup canned or frozen corn
⅓ cup cooked basmati rice

Put the chicken in a saucepan together with the bay leaf, parsley, and peppercorns and pour in the stock. Bring to a boil, then cover and simmer gently for 40 minutes or until the chicken is tender and cooked through.

Remove the chicken from the bone and chop into small pieces. Strain the stock and reserve. Melt the butter in a pan, stir in the flour, and cook for 1 minute. Gradually whisk in the stock, bring to a boil, and then cook for 1 minute. Stir in the corn and continue to cook for a couple of minutes. Mix together the chopped chicken, rice, stock, and corn. Puree the mixture for younger babies.

Creamy chicken and vegetables

🍼 9–12 MONTHS

🥣 MAKES 3 PORTIONS

🕐 COOKING TIME: 17 MINUTES

❄ SUITABLE FOR FREEZING

1 tablespoon vegetable oil
½ cup chopped onion
2 medium carrots, peeled and chopped
¾ cup wiped and sliced button mushrooms
1 tablespoon all-purpose flour
½ cup Chicken Stock (see page 125)
¼ cup milk
½ cup chopped cooked chicken
¼ cup grated Cheddar cheese

Using leftover roast chicken, this makes a nutritious and tasty dish for your baby. If you don't have any cooked chicken, poach half a chicken breast in some chicken stock for about 6 minutes or until cooked through.

Heat the oil in a saucepan and sauté the onion and carrots for 5 minutes, stirring occasionally. Add the mushrooms and sauté for 3 minutes. Stir in the flour and continue to cook for 1 minute. Gradually stir in the stock and the milk. Bring to a boil, then lower the heat and cook for 5 minutes. Stir in the chicken and cook for 1 more minute. Remove from the heat and stir in the cheese until melted. Either chop into small pieces or puree for your baby.

This tasty recipe will help encourage your baby to enjoy eating red meat.

My first spaghetti Bolognese

1½ tablespoons vegetable oil
1 clove garlic, crushed
½ cup chopped onion
1 medium carrot, peeled and grated
¾ cup wiped and sliced button mushrooms
5 ounces lean ground beef
½ cup canned crushed tomatoes
1 cup Chicken Stock (see page 125)
A few drops of Worcestershire sauce
Pinch of brown sugar
1 bay leaf
2 ounces spaghetti

Heat 1 tablespoon of the oil in a saucepan and sauté the garlic and onion for 2 minutes. Add the grated carrot and sauté for 2 minutes more. Pour in the remaining oil and sauté the mushrooms for about 3 minutes.

Meanwhile, sauté the ground beef in a dry frying pan until browned, then add to the vegetables together with the tomatoes, stock, Worcestershire sauce, sugar, and bay leaf. Cover the saucepan and simmer for about 15 minutes; remove bay leaf. Cook the spaghetti according to the package instructions, but do not add salt.

Puree the cooked meat using a handheld electric blender for a smoother texture. Chop up the spaghetti into short lengths and stir into the Bolognese sauce.

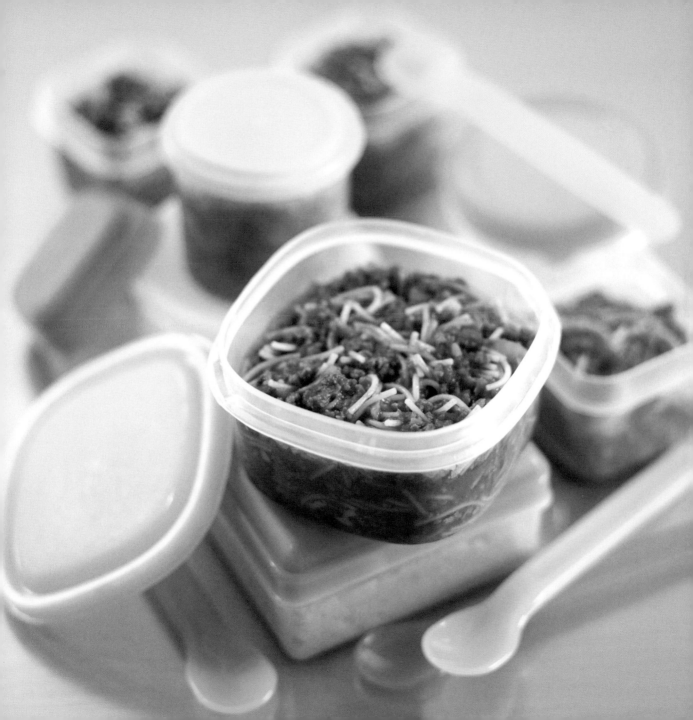

The onion and carrots in this recipe give the beef a wonderful flavor, and the long, slow cooking makes it beautifully tender.

TOP TIP
If your baby doesn't like eating meat, you need to ensure that she's getting enough iron, so include foods in her diet like lentils, dark green leafy vegetables, and fortified breakfast cereals.

Old-fashioned beef casserole

1 onion, sliced
1½ tablespoons vegetable oil
8 ounces lean stewing beef, cut into chunks
2 medium carrots, peeled and sliced
3 medium potatoes (12 ounces), peeled and diced
1 tablespoon chopped fresh parsley
2 cups Chicken Stock (see page 125)

Preheat the oven to 300°F. Sauté the onion in the vegetable oil in a casserole dish until lightly golden. Add the beef and sauté until browned. Add the carrots, potatoes, and parsley, pour in the stock, and bring the mixture to a boil. Cover, transfer the casserole to the oven, and cook for about 2 hours or until the meat is really tender (adding extra stock if necessary). Chop into small pieces or, for younger babies, blend to a puree of the desired consistency.

Tender casserole of lamb

9–12 MONTHS

MAKES 4 PORTIONS

COOKING TIME: 1 HOUR

SUITABLE FOR FREEZING

Two 2- to 3-ounce lamb chops
½ small onion, chopped
2 medium potatoes (8 ounces), peeled and diced
2 medium carrots, peeled and sliced
2 medium tomatoes (8 ounces), peeled, seeded,
and chopped (see page 126)
½ cup Chicken Stock (see page 125)

Preheat the oven to 350°F. Put the lamb, vegetables, and stock into a small casserole, cover, and bake for about 1 hour or until the lamb is tender. Chop into small pieces, or puree for younger babies.

Cooking lamb in a casserole with vegetables and stock makes it sufficiently tender and moist for your baby.

TOP TIP
Once your baby starts feeding herself, you may find that mealtimes take a lot longer, so try to allow for this.

This dish makes a great way to start the day. Serve it as it is or mix with some yogurt.

TOP TIP
Never leave your baby alone while she is eating. Sometimes babies try to swallow food without chewing it and choking can be a real hazard. If your baby chokes, do not try to fish the food from the back of her mouth, as you may only end up pushing it farther down her throat. Tip her face-down over your lap with her head lower than her stomach and slap her firmly between the shoulder blades to dislodge the food. If the food is coughed up into her mouth, carefully remove it.

Fruity muesli

1 cup rolled oats
¼ cup wheat germ
¼ cup chopped dried apricots
½ cup orange juice
1 apple, peeled and grated

Mix the oats together with the wheat germ and apricots. Pour in the orange juice and leave to soak for at least 5 minutes. Stir in the grated apple and blitz for a few seconds using a handheld electric blender.

The secret of a good old-fashioned rice pudding is long, slow, gentle cooking.

Traditional rice pudding

1 tablespoon butter, plus extra for greasing
3½ tablespoons long-grain rice (not converted)
2 tablespoons light brown or superfine sugar
2 cups milk
1 vanilla bean or ½ teaspoon pure vanilla extract

Preheat the oven to 300°F. Grease a shallow ovenproof dish with a little butter. Put the rice and sugar into the dish and pour in the milk. Split the vanilla bean (if using) and scrape the seeds into the dish, or add the vanilla extract and dot with the butter. Bake for about 2 hours, stirring occasionally. Serve warm and mix with some fruit, raisins, or one of the choices below.

Good things to serve with rice pudding:
- stewed apple and pear
- canned peaches
- chopped mango
- strawberry jam
- golden syrup
- fruit compote

This is a quicker version of making rice pudding, cooking it on top of the stove rather than in the oven.

TOP TIP
After the age of one year, if your child is fussy and eats only a small variety of foods, continuing with standard infant formula milk or next-step formula (targeted at babies over one) milk instead of using cow's milk might be beneficial.

Quick rice pudding

3½ tablespoons long-grain rice (not converted)
2 cups milk
1 to 2 tablespoons superfine sugar
½ teaspoon pure vanilla extract

Put the rice, milk, sugar, and vanilla in a heavy-bottomed saucepan. Bring to a boil, then reduce the heat, cover, and simmer for 30 to 35 minutes, stirring occasionally. Mix with fruit or one of the toppings from Traditional Rice Pudding (see page 119).

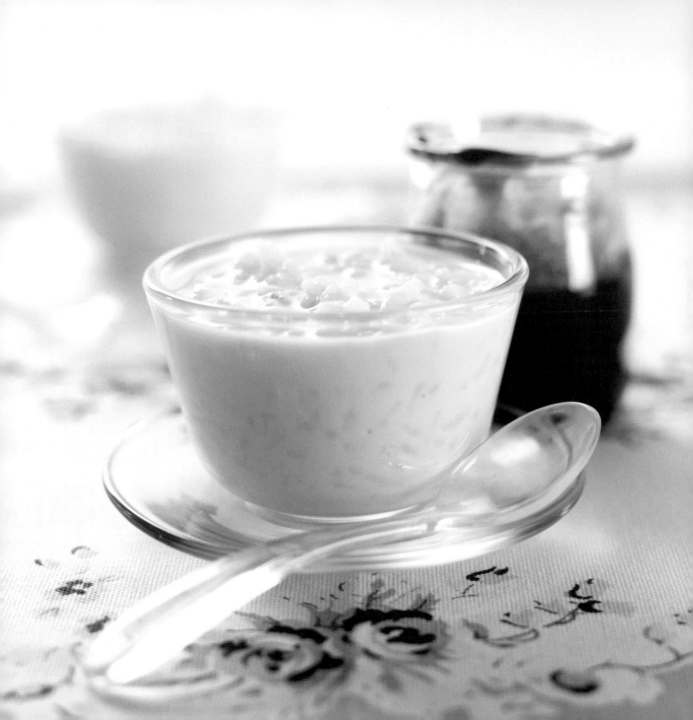

9–12 MONTHS

MAKES 2 PORTIONS

COOKING TIME: 7–8 MINUTES

SUITABLE FOR FREEZING

This dish is good on its own, or you could mix the fruit with yogurt or stir into rice pudding.

Nectarine and strawberry with vanilla

2 nectarines or peaches, peeled, pitted, and chopped
(see page 126)
⅓ cup hulled and quartered strawberries
1 vanilla bean

Put the nectarines and strawberries into a heavy-bottomed saucepan. Split the vanilla bean and, using a sharp knife, scrape out the seeds and add to the fruit together with the bean. Cover and cook over low heat for 7 to 8 minutes. Remove the vanilla bean and mash or chop the fruit.

9–12 MONTHS

MAKES 1 PORTION

COOKING TIME: 2 MINUTES

UNSUITABLE FOR FREEZING

Bananas are easy to digest and provide a good source of energy for your baby.

Yummy banana

1 tablespoon unsalted butter
1 small banana, sliced
3 tablespoons orange juice

Melt the butter in a small frying pan or saucepan and sauté the banana for 1 minute. Pour in the orange juice and cook for another minute. Mash with a fork.

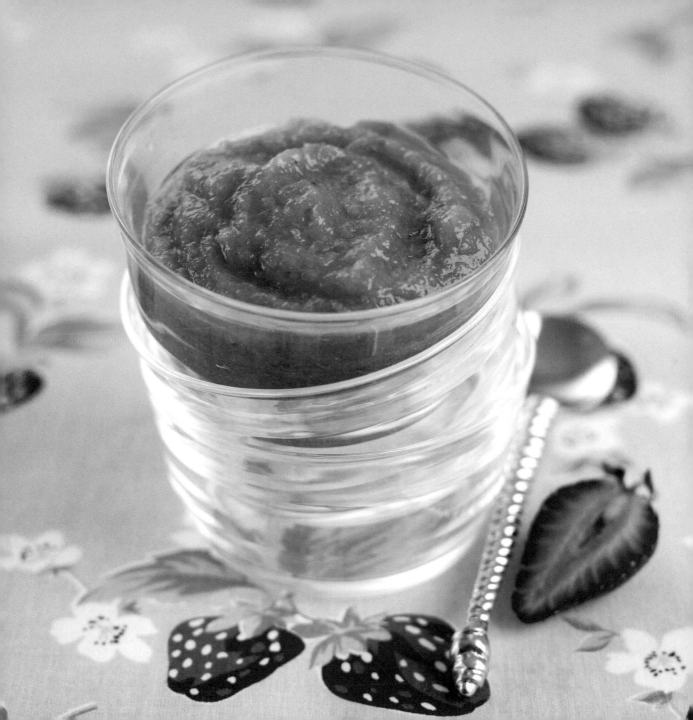

Basics

Vegetable stock

6 MONTHS +

MAKES 2 CUPS

COOKING TIME:
1 HOUR 7 MINS

SUITABLE FOR FREEZING
BUT NOT SUITABLE FOR
REFREEZING IN A PUREE

It is best to use homemade stock when cooking for a young baby, as stock cubes are high in salt and therefore unsuitable for babies under a year. In addition, it is important to use fresh and not previously frozen stock when making baby purees that you intend to freeze. Vegetable stock is very easy to make and will keep in the fridge for up to a week.

1 onion
1 clove garlic
2 large carrots, peeled
1 large leek, washed
1 stalk celery, trimmed
1 tablespoon olive oil
3½ cups cold water
1 bouquet garni or a mixture of fresh herbs (e.g., sprig
    of thyme, parsley, and oregano, and a bay leaf)
4 black peppercorns

Roughly chop all the vegetables. Heat the oil in a large, heavy-bottomed saucepan and sauté the onion and garlic for 2 minutes. Add the rest of the vegetables and cook over low heat for 5 minutes to soften in the oil without browning, covering if you like.

Pour in the water and bring to a boil, then add the bouquet garni and peppercorns. Reduce the heat, cover, and simmer for 1 hour.

Leave to cool for about 2 hours, then strain through a sieve. Squeeze the remaining juices out of the vegetables by pushing them down in the sieve with a potato masher.

Chicken stock

Carcass from a roast chicken or about 2 pounds
*   chicken bones, chopped into pieces*
3 large carrots, peeled
1 parsnip, peeled
1 large leek, washed
2 onions
1 stalk celery, trimmed
Small bunch of parsley
Sprig of thyme
1 bay leaf
4 black peppercorns
8 cups boiling water

Put the carcass into a large, heavy-bottomed saucepan. Roughly chop all the vegetables and add to the pan together with the herbs and peppercorns. Pour in the water, bring to a boil, and then remove all the surface sediment with a slotted spoon. Half cover the pan and simmer gently for 1½ hours or until the liquid is reduced by half.

Allow to cool, then leave in the fridge overnight. Remove any congealed fat from the top in the morning. Strain the chicken and vegetables to make the stock.

6 MONTHS +

MAKES 6 CUPS

COOKING TIME: 1½ HOURS

SUITABLE FOR FREEZING BUT NOT SUITABLE FOR REFREEZING IN A PUREE

Making your own chicken stock sounds laborious, but it is actually very easy. Simply take the carcass from a roast chicken to form the basis of your stock or use some chicken bones. The stock will keep in the fridge for 3 days.

Basic cheese sauce

1 tablespoon unsalted butter
1 tablespoon all-purpose flour
1 cup milk
⅓ cup grated Cheddar cheese

Melt the butter in a saucepan, stir in the flour to make a smooth paste, and cook for 1 minute. Gradually stir in the milk, bring to a boil, and cook for a few minutes over low heat until thickened and smooth. Stir in the grated cheese until melted.

Peeling tomatoes and peaches/nectarines

Plunge the tomatoes in boiling water for 30 seconds. Transfer to cold water, then peel, seed, and chop. For peaches/nectarines, score a cross on the base of each fruit, then submerge in boiling water for 1 minute. Peel, cut in half, discarding the pit, and chop the flesh.

Index

Page numbers in **bold** indicate a recipe where the entry is a main ingredient.

allergies 7, 9, 12–17
apples **25**, **26–7**, **50–1**, **54**, 57, **60–1**, 81, **90**, **95**
apricots 17, 38, 39, **61–2**, **91**
avocados 30, **31**, **55**
baby rice cereal 9, 10, 13, 18
bananas 9, 30, **31**, **52–5**, 56, **87**, **92–3**, **95**, **122**
beef **84**, **85**, **114–15**, **116**
blueberries **54**, **59**, **95**
breast milk 7, 8–9, 13, 14, 17, 18
broccoli **28**, 34, 45, 68, **72–3**, **105**
butternut squash 28–9, 42, 43, **74**
carrots **22–3**, 40, 41, **46–7**, 65, 67, 70, **76–7**, **82–3**, **85**, **99**, **105**
cauliflower 34, **67**, 70, **72–3**
cheese 10, 33, **48–9**, 70, **71**, **72–3**, **74**, **76–7**, **98**, **99**, **105**, 108, 126
    cheese sauce **126**
cherries **92–3**
chicken **50–1**, **58**, 80, 81, **82–3**, **110**, **111**, **112**, **113**
    chicken stock **125**
choking 118
constipation 108
corn 34, **46–7**, 80, 112
corn on the cob **34**
cow's milk protein allergies 14–15
dairy products 7, 97
    allergies to 14–15
eczema 17
eggs 9, 12, 63, **98**
    allergies to 16
fat in the diet 70
fibrous foods 7
finger foods 63, 97
fish 9, 12, **48–9**, **75**, **76–7**, **78–9**, 108

food additives and colorings 17
food intolerance 13
food mill 11
foods to avoid 9–10
formula milk 7, 8, 14, 18
freezing food 11
fruit 7–8, 11, **24**, **25**, **38–9**, 63
fruity muesli **118**
gluten 10, 16
honey 9
iron-rich foods 7, 8, 19, 33, 63, 111
kiwifruit 33
lactose intolerance 15
lamb **86**, **117**
leeks 65, **82–3**
lentils **64**
mangoes 38, **54**, **55**, **91**
meat, red 33, 63, 84, 85
melon 38, **54**
microwaving 10, 12
milk 7, 8–9
    allergies 12, 13, 14–15
muesli **87**, **118**
nectarines 39, **122–3**, 126
no-cook purees 30–1, 52–5
nutritional needs of babies 7–8
nuts 9, 12
oatmeal **88–9**
oats **87**, **88–9**, 90
papayas 9, **31**, **54**
parsnips 37, **85**
pasta **74**, **102–3**, **104**, **106–7**, **109**, **111**, **114–15**
peaches 39, **54**, 56, **57**, **59**, **95**, 126
peanut allergies 16
pears **25**, **26–7**, **55**, **57**, **59**, **60–1**, **90**, **95**
peas **37**, **40**, 42, 45, 65, 68, **82–3**
pineapple 33
plums 39
potatoes 10, **42**, **46–7**, 65, **105**

preterm babies 18–19
prunes **90**
pumpkin **43**
pureeing 11
reheating food 12
rice 9, 10, 13, 18, **97**, **98**, **99**, **110**, **112**, **119**, **120–1**,
root vegetables 9, 13, **29**
rutabaga 37, **40**
salt 10
seeds 9, 12
shellfish 9, 12
solids, starting 7, 23
soups **69**, **80**
soy products 14–15
spinach 37, **45**, 68, **108**
steaming 10–11
stewing fruit 11
stocks **124–5**
strawberries **54**, 57, **95**, **122**, **123**
sugar 10
sweet potatoes **28**, 37, **42**, 45, **50–1**, **85**, **86**
tofu, banana with 55
tomatoes 37, **66–7**, 70, **74**, **76–7**, **99**, **104**, **109**, **110**, 126
tooth decay 56
tuna **97**
vanilla **60–1**, **122–3**
vegetables 7–8, 9, 10–11, **22–3**, **24**, **34–7**, **48–9**, 63, 70, **71**, 81, **106–7**, 113
    vegetable stock **124**; see also root vegetables
vegetarian babies 64, 71
vitamin supplements 8
water 46
wheat-based foods 10, 12
yogurt 33, **55**
zucchini **34**, **42**, 68, **70**

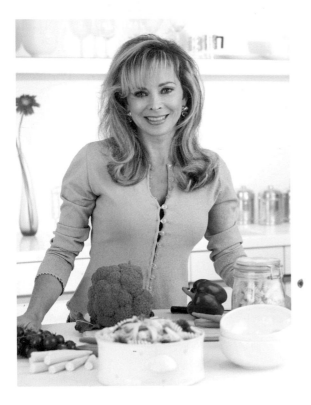

Acknowledgments

I would like to thank the following for their help on this book:
Sarah Lavelle, Dave King, Kate Parker, Caroline King, Dr. Jane Morgan, Dr. Mary Fewtrell, Dagmar Vesely, Jo Harris, Carey Smith, Katherine Hockley, Dr. Michel Cohen, Judith Curr, Greer Hendricks, Suzanne O'Neill, Sybil Pincus, Virginia McRae, and all at Smith & Gilmour. Thanks also to the mothers and babies who feature in the book: Claire and Leo Bowers, Helena and Tomas Caldon, Beverley and Chase Calvert, Laura and Charlie Davies, Rosie and Maia Hallam, Daniella and Luca Pillitto, and Julie and Emily Zimmerman.

About the Author

Annabel Karmel is a leading author on cooking for children and has written twelve bestselling books that are sold all over the world. After the tragic loss of her first child, who died of a rare viral disease at just three months, Annabel wrote her first book, *The Complete Baby and Toddler Meal Planner*, now an international bestseller. A mother of three, she is an expert at devising tasty and nutritious meals for children without the need for parents to spend hours in the kitchen. Annabel writes regularly for national newspapers and appears frequently on television as the top expert on children's nutritional issues. She travels frequently to the United States, where she has published *The Healthy Baby Meal Planner, First Meals, Mom and Me Cookbook,* and *Favorite Family Meals*. For more recipes and information, go to www.annabelkarmel.com.

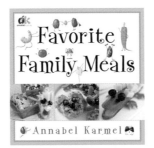

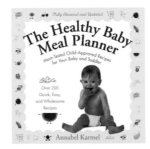